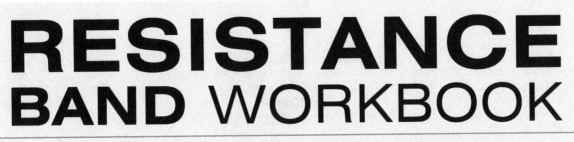

RESISTANCE
BAND WORKBOOK

Illustrated Step-by-Step Guide to Stretching, Strengthening and Rehabilitative Techniques

Dr. Karl Knopf

T0061970

ULYSSES PRESS

Published in the United States by
Ulysses Press
P.O. Box 3440
Berkeley, CA 94703
www.ulyssespress.com

ISBN: 978-1-61243-171-0
Library of Congress Control Number 2013931801

Printed in the United States

10 9 8

Acquisitions: Kelly Reed
Managing editor: Claire Chun
Editor: Lily Chou
Proofreader: Elyce Berrigan-Dunlop
Indexer: Sayre Van Young
Front cover design: what!design @ whatweb.com
Photographs: © Rapt Productions
Models: Mary J. Gines, Chris Knopf, Karl Knopf, Toni Silver

Please Note

RESISTANCE
BAND WORKBOOK

contents

PART 1

overview

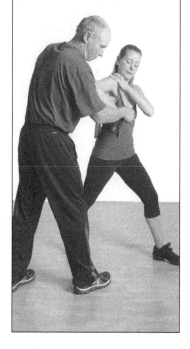

introduction

Welcome to the world of resistance bands! Resistance training bands were ranked with stability balls as the most popular piece of exercise equipment in a 2011 IDEA Personal Training Equipment Trends report. Resistance tubing and bands are popular because they're lightweight and easy to transport, which means they can be used when traveling. Many trainers and therapists like the band because they can adapt any exercise to a functional application.

These latex training devices have been around since the 1970s, yet they're a mainstay of almost every fitness enthusiast. Bands were first used in therapy to introduce low-intensity resistance to rehabilitating patients. Today bands come in all shapes and resistances and can be used by people of all ages and fitness levels.

Resistance Band Workbook features almost every conceivable exercise ever done with an exercise band. Whether you're looking to enhance your physique, elevate your sports performance or simply improve functional fitness, this book will add a new dimension to your workout—regardless of your experience level with resistance training.

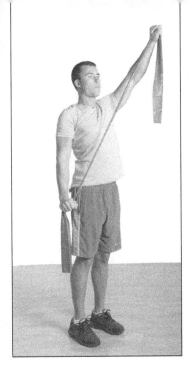

what is resistance training?

Chances are you're familiar with the term "strength training." You might also know about— and even perform—weightlifting, weight training, resistance training or progressive resistance exercise. Simply put, these terms are used interchangeably by the public to describe the act of harnessing a resistance to place a load/strain on a muscle to develop muscle or improve muscular endurance.

Strength training can take many forms, from lifting your own body against the resistance of gravity to using weights or exercise bands to challenge your muscles. It really doesn't matter what shape or form the resistance comes in because the ultimate goal is to improve strength, muscle size (hypertrophy), muscular endurance or power.

The best method to improve strength is often referred to as progressive resistance exercise training. Here, a person engages in a set of exercises that slowly and progressively overload a muscle. When the muscle adapts to the challenge of a load/resistance and the resistance becomes easier, the person either increases the resistance/load or performs more repetitions. The general rule of thumb is when you can perform 10–15 reps easily and correctly, you need to increase the load. In weight training you increase the weight, but in resistance band training you progress to the next harder band or combine two bands together.

As you improve in strength, it's advised to increase the volume of work you perform by adding "sets" to your workout. Two to three sets of each exercise are ideal.

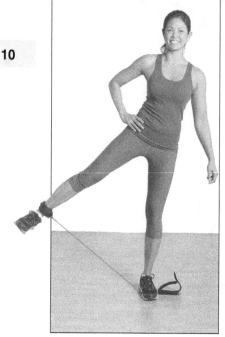

why train with bands?

The adaptability and versatility of resistance training bands make them suitable for all levels, from those recovering from injury to world-class athletes. In addition, the beauty of performing resistance band training is that you don't need to buy or store heavy equipment or drive to a gym. Every exercise that can be done on a piece of exercise equipment or with weights can be done with an exercise band.

There may be even more opportunities with band training than with weight training. The bands come in varying resistances, so as you get stronger you can purchase heavier-resistance bands in order to accommodate your improvements in strength. They can be easily and quickly exchanged to increase or decrease the resistance depending upon the exercise. You can also exercise a muscle at various angles as well as both eccentrically and concentrically. A total-body resistance band workout should take less than 15 minutes and can be done practically anywhere—even in the pool.

Here are additional benefits of training with bands:

- Increased strength in muscles and bones
- Improved balance
- Reduced lower back pain
- Improved blood sugar control
- Improved blood transport system
- Increased metabolism
- Reduced arthritic pain

Just keep in mind that exercise bands alone will not offer great changes in muscular hypertrophy, or massive muscle development, but for most people band training provides adequate results. The band is versatile and convenient, and it tones the muscles with low risk of injury. However, be aware that you may compromise the quality of your training by incorrectly placing your hands on the bands or allowing the band to control the movement.

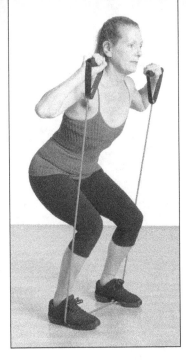

choosing a band

Resistance bands are typically made of latex and come in several shapes and intensities. They're commercially available at most sporting goods stores and therapy outlets and through online vendors. Selecting the correct band for your goals and body type is critical for obtaining ideal results. Ultimately, through personal trial and error you'll determine which shape and style works best for you and your objective.

Today manufacturers produce exercise bands that accommodate every level of ability. Depending on the manufacturer, the color of the band generally denotes the intensity. Usually a light color such as pink and yellow is the easiest resistance, green and red moderate and dark gray and black very intense. However, please keep in mind that no standards exist between band manufacturers (one manufacturer's pink band may be much harder than another manufacturer's pink band) so select the band you use based on how it feels rather than the color.

There are basically two forms of resistance bands: flat and tubular. The flat one is the most common and is available latex-free for those with a latex allergy. Sometimes bands come in rolls and can be cut for specific purposes; they can also be purchased pre-cut. Most exercises can be completed with a three- to six-foot piece of band; you can "choke up" on the band to make it fit your needs. If you've never used bands before, start with the flat band and progress from there.

The tubular version is becoming more popular because it's more durable and comes with padded handles. You may even find tubing with adjustable handles in order to adapt the length of the tubing to the individual. However, you can purchase handles for the flat variety. Wrapping the flat band around a small piece of PVC pipe can also provide a wonderful handle. Some resistance training bands are loops that can be wrapped around your limbs to provide additional challenges. You may also come across a figure eight-shaped exercise band, an exercise bar and a braided exercise tube. Some of these bands can

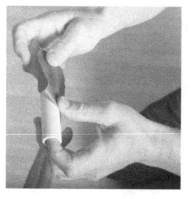
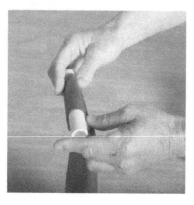

Band wrapped around PVC pipe

be attached to free weights to increase resistance, which introduces additional training elements to an exercise, such as improving control and decreasing unwanted momentum in explosive maneuvers.

In general, all the exercises in this book can be done with either type of band. However, if you're just looking for an overall muscular toning routine, the flat band works very well. The flat version can also be rolled up easily and transported.

Even more options exist, such as attachments that secure the band to a wall, your ankle or your thigh. Some manufacturers sell variable bands with brackets that attach securely and safely to a closed door and have three levels of bands attached with upper and lower handles.

Keep in mind, however, that both types of bands will deteriorate over time. Exposure to the elements and hand oils accelerate the process. Therefore, it's wise to regularly review the status of your band.

The implementation of bands is limitless. While all these options are nice, they're by no means critical to get an ideal workout. If you do use these, always double-check that the band won't come loose when you apply force.

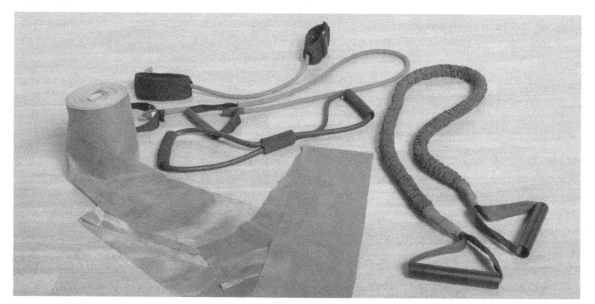

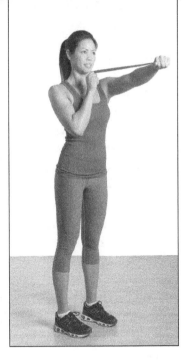

before you begin

Engaging in a resistance training program is generally a very safe way to participate in growing stronger. While resistance band training is considered safe, always train smart to prevent injuries or increased joint discomfort and muscle soreness. Try your best to execute each rep with the best form possible to avoid any discomfort and to obtain the best results.

As with any form of exercise, it's wise to consult your health provider before starting an exercise program to make sure the program is suited to your particular goals and health concerns. In Part 2 (see page 15) you'll find sample programs designed for specific goals. You might also have your health provider review the programs and tweak them specifically for your concerns.

Exercise bands can be used by everyone. If you have a serious joint condition, practice the moves without bands for one to two weeks to commit the movement to your muscle memory.

If you can perform the moves without any increase in pain, then introduce the lightest band into the program. Always keep in mind the two-hour rule: Two hours post-exercise, you should not experience increased pain. While slight muscle soreness might be expected, a significant increase in joint or muscle pain means that the way you're performing the exercise or the intensity of the band being used needs to be re-assessed. You may need to select another exercise that addresses that muscle group or joint area.

Matching the correct band resistance to each exercise is critical. Most people use the same band for all exercises, which is OK. However, using a lighter band for isolated exercises such as triceps exercises and a heavier band for compound exercises such as chest presses is ideal.

Perfect posture is also important for a good, safe training session. When sitting, sit on your "sit bones," which are the tips of your pelvis, not your tailbone; your feet should provide additional support. Be sure to sit tall—don't slouch.

When standing, engage in proper neutral spine posture. From a side view, your ears should be stacked over your shoulders, shoul-

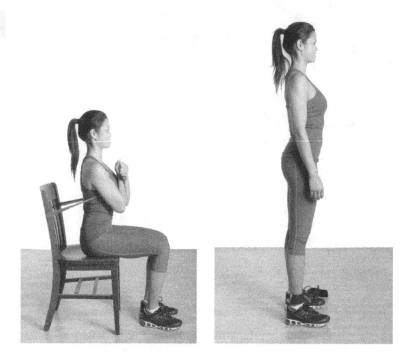

Good posture sitting (top) and standing (bottom)

ders over hips and hips over ankles. Your weight should be evenly distributed over both feet and your knees are softly bent; your hips should neither tilt upward or downward. Keep your chest high without arching your back.

Here are 10 tips to a safe, effective and successful workout:

- Make sure you're healthy enough to perform the exercise. Don't make pain!

- Always prepare the body for resistance training by performing a complete warm-up.
- Always execute the movement with proper posture and with sound biomechanics. Don't sacrifice form to do sloppy repetitions.
- Never hold your breath. Holding your breath can increase your blood pressure and cause dizziness and other ill effects.

Exhale on the hardest part of the exercise and inhale on the return portion.

- Listen to your body. If your shoulder is bothering you one day, skip the shoulder exercises but train the other parts of the body instead. If you experience pain, stop. If you have pain two hours post-exercise, re-evaluate the exercise and the intensity of the band.
- Be regular—ideally aim to perform some form of strength training two to three times a week.
- Perform the exercise through the full range of motion.
- Perform the movements slowly and with control—don't allow the band to snap back. You control the band; don't let the band control you.
- Check the exercise band periodically for wear.
- Train, don't strain. It's OK to back off, but don't quit.

PART 2

the
programs

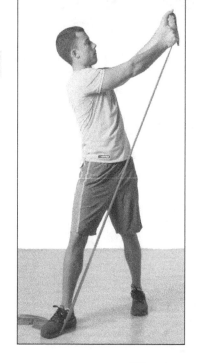

how to use this book

This section of *Resistance Band Workbook* presents programs for a wide range of sports and orthopedic issues. Pick the one that best suits your needs, or use these samples as a springboard to create your own routine. The sample routines are designed so that you start with basic moves and progress to more advanced ones. The exercises are grouped by target body area.

Before you jump into your resistance training workout, remember to warm up to prepare your body for exercise. A warm-up can consist of light aerobic activity that limbers up the muscles you plan to engage. It can also be a very light version of the exercise you plan to perform. The best method is to combine the two, doing a few minutes of aerobic exercise to warm up the body and then a light set of each exercise before you do your more formal sets. (See page 105 for warm-up suggestions.) The American College of Sports Medicine and the American Heart Association suggest we need to do at least 30 minutes of aerobic exercise three to five times a week, and strength training two to three times a week. While you can do band work anytime, many people find it best to do their band training after their aerobic exercise, followed by a stretching session.

As you do your resistance band exercises, never sacrifice quality for quantity. Perform each repetition in a smooth and controlled manner; work your joints through their full range of motion. It's generally recommended that the difficult (concentric) aspect of the move should take 2–3 seconds to perform, while the easy (eccentric) part should take equally as long. The bottom line is that you control the band; don't allow the band to control you. In addition, don't do the move super slowly or too quickly. Note also that most exercises can be done from sitting or standing depending on your preference.

Beginners should choose a band that enables them to do at least one set of 8 reps; follow this procedure for one to two weeks. After two weeks, consider adding a second set. It's best to do one set, rest for 45 seconds, and then do another set of the same exercise. When you can do two sets of 8 reps without straining, it's time to add just enough resistance so that it's difficult to do 6–8 reps. From here, work yourself back up to 8–15 reps. Add resistance in small increments. If you're not ready to progress to the next-level band, try putting two easy bands together. Keep in mind that the more fit you are, the slower the gains will be when compared to a beginner. Remember, you're NOT competing with anyone. Don't let anyone "should" on you.

Those at the intermediate and advanced levels should select a band resistance that best matches their goals. The number of sets and reps are also determined by this. The general rule of thumb is low reps of higher intensity for strength and hypertrophy and high reps for muscular endurance. Train smart to avoid injury. Keep in mind that it's always important to prepare the joint for activity. Unfortunately, the more advanced you are, the more likely you are to skip the joint preparation aspect of your routine, and probably even skip the stretching at the end. Please don't skip either aspect because oftentimes skipping over them leads to issues down the road.

After your workout, a cool-down period is prudent. This allows your body to taper off from your workout—you don't want to stop abruptly. Spend 5–15 minutes stretching the muscles you engaged in your workout. Turn to page 105 for some safe and effective stretches.

Bands with Balls & Bells

Adding bands to a weight-training routine provides an isokinetic resistance, keeping the motion smoother and not jerky, which is common in some weight-training exercises. The dumbbell-and-band series is for those who are extremely experienced with band training and wish to challenge their workout. It's best to use a flat band that can be wrapped around the dumbbell handles rather than using exercise bands with handles. Some trainers like to use the bands with handles, but you might find it much easier to position everything when using a flat band. These exercises are more strenuous so be sure to use proper breathing patterns.

Advanced practitioners can also incorporate some exercises while using a stability ball. The value of performing the moves on a ball is that this requires further concentration and engages the total body in the movement. It's important to note that a lighter resistance should be used in this scenario.

Designing a Resistance Band Training Program

After you've followed the sample workouts for a while, you may want to create your own resistance band program. Aim to make it fun with the purpose of improving your function. Only you know what's important to you and what you enjoy. It's suggested that you change the program every three months or so to exercise the muscles in a different fashion. Too often people who exercise overwork certain areas, which leads to injury and postural imbalances. A simple assessment you can perform is to look at yourself in the mirror. If your shoulders are rounded, do more upper back exercises and so on.

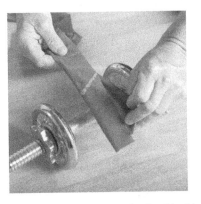
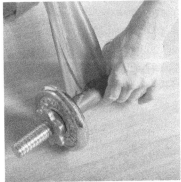

Wrapping a band around a dumbbell handle

The first step in designing a safe and sane strength-training program is to cater to your particular health status and personal goals. Pay special attention to any health issues or painful joint areas. It's wise to solicit input from your health professional about any precautions and recommendations. It's also critical that you understand the concept of dose and response. Too much "dose" causes a bad response (discomfort and injury); too little dose causes no response and thus no benefits.

Each workout should not exceed 12 exercises and should engage all the major muscles of the body. If you choose to do more sets, then decrease the number of exercises. Another thing to consider is that if, for example, you do a great deal of walking or biking, then spend the majority of your band program on body parts not addressed in other aspects of your training. The goal of any training program is to have a balanced routine.

Deciding on which exercises to include is much like selecting which wine you'll pair with your meal—it's a little bit of science and a little bit of art. My suggestion is start out with one exercise for your chest and pair it with an exercise for your upper back. Then include an exercise for your biceps (front of the upper arm) and pair it with a triceps exercise (back of the upper arm). Do something for your shoulders, then move to the lower body and do something for the front of the leg matched with an exercise for the back of the leg. Finish it off with a core exercise. Anything more than that is dessert.

Aim to do 8–15 repetitions per set. However, when doing band training, going too fast is just wasting your time. The more reps you perform, the more focus you place on muscular endurance. Choosing a heavier band and doing lower reps emphasizes strength and power. Try to do at least 2–3 sets of each exercise. Another option is just exercise for 30 seconds then rest for 10 seconds.

When you reach a plateau and stop seeing improvement, it's a good time to tweak your routine by changing the exercises or the number of reps and/or sets. Athletes may even take a week off or change their routine completely. It's also perfectly fine to change your workout (for instance, switch out one chest exercise for another) if you get bored. Your exercise program is a living document that will need to be adapted approximately every three to four months.

Level 1: Getting Started

This program is designed to acquaint you and your body with resistance band exercises. While it may appear basic, it's comprehensive, addressing the major muscle groups of the body, and could be a mainstay routine. Focus on staying mindful of perfect form, proper body mechanics and correct breathing.

LEVEL 1: GETTING STARTED

Warm up for at least 10 minutes. See pages 105–12 for suggestions.

EXERCISE	SETS	REP/TIME	REST
Pull-Down p. 45	1	8–15	30–45 sec
Horizontal Chest Press p. 48	1	8–15	30–45 sec
Reverse Flye p. 47	1	8–15	30–45 sec
Frontal Raise p. 50	1	8–15	30–45 sec
Horizontal Triceps Extension p. 60	1	8–15	30–45 sec
Biceps Curl p. 65	1	8–15	30–45 sec
Gas Pedal p. 70	1	8–15	30–45 sec
Leg Press p. 71	1	8–15	30–45 sec

Level 2: Growing Strong

This program is an excellent way to tone and strengthen the entire body in a short amount of time. Increasing the reps and resistance level will keep you strong and toned forever.

LEVEL 2: GROWING STRONG

Warm up for at least 10 minutes. See pages 105–12 for suggestions.

EXERCISE	SETS	REP/TIME	REST
Long Row *p. 55*	2	6–8	30–45 sec
Shoulder Press *p. 52*	2	6–8	30–45 sec
Biceps Curl *p. 65*	2	6–8	30–45 sec
Triceps Extension *p. 59*	2	6–8	30–45 sec
Trombone Press *p.63*	2	6–8	30–45 sec
Squat *p. 72*	2	6–8	30–45 sec
Forward Lunge *p. 74*	2	6–8	30–45 sec
Reverse Wood Chop *p. 81*	2	6–8	30–45 sec

Level 3: Advanced

This program is designed for those who have the time to concentrate on taking their workout to the next level. Start out by following the program listed here. As you advance in strength and ability, attach a band to your strength-training equipment such as a dumbbell or exercise bar, to perform dual-resistance exercises. Doing dumbbell-and-band exercises is an extra challenge and also really fun. Again, this is only for the super-advanced and should be done with a spotter nearby until you're proficient. Make sure the ball will support you and any extra load.

LEVEL 3: ADVANCED

Warm up for at least 10 minutes. See pages 105–12 for suggestions.

EXERCISE	SETS	REP/TIME	REST
Incline Chest Press *p. 49*	3	8–15	30–45 sec
Flye *p. 46*	3	8–15	30–45 sec
Lateral Raise *p. 51*	3	8–15	30–45 sec
Upright Row *p. 56*	3	8–15	30–45 sec
Shoulder Press *p. 52*	3	8–15	30–45 sec
Chest Press on Ball *p. 96*	3	8–15	30–45 sec
Biceps Curl *p. 65*	3	8–15	30–45 sec
Reverse Curl *p. 66*	3	8–15	30–45 sec
Push-Up *p. 85*	3	8–15	30–45 sec
Lawnmower Pull *p. 62*	3	8–15	30–45 sec
Attachment Leg Abduction *p. 91*	3	8–15	30–45 sec
Attachment Leg Adduction *p. 92*	3	8–15	30–45 sec
Half Sit-Up *p. 80*	3	8–15	30–45 sec

This workout is designed expressly for highly fit folks who desire to push their fitness level to new heights. Don't perform this workout if you have any health issues or are afraid of a little pain and discomfort. This routine is not intended to be done more than once a week.

SUPER-FIT

Warm up for at least 10 minutes. See pages 105–12 for suggestions.

EXERCISE	SETS	REP/TIME	REST
Squat *p. 72*	3	8–15	30–60 sec
Squat Shuffle *p. 73*	3	8–15	30–60 sec
Forward Lunge *p. 74*	3	8–15	30–60 sec
Leg Abduction *p. 77*	3	8–15	30–45 sec
Side Step *p. 75*	3	8–15	30–60 sec
Reverse Wood Chop *p. 81*	3	8–15	30–60 sec
Attachment Long Row *p. 88*	3	8–15	30–60 sec
Attachment Torso Rotation *p. 95*	3	8–15	30–60 sec
Chair Dip *p. 61*	3	8–15	30–60 sec
Push-Up *p. 85*	3	8–15	30–60 sec
Dual-Resistance Chest Press *p. 100*	3	8–15	30–60 sec
Dual-Resistance Chest Flye *p. 101*	3	8–15	30–60 sec
Dual-Resistance Lateral Raise *p. 102*	3	8–15	30–60 sec
Dual-Resistance Frontal Raise *p. 103*	3	8–15	30–60 sec
Dual-Resistance Biceps Curl *p. 104*	3	8–15	30–60 sec

Baseball/Softball

Baseball and softball can be played competitively or recreationally, with each position requiring a different level of fitness. Anyone who has ever played either sport knows how important shoulder flexibility and core strength are. This workout is a general, overall routine.

BASEBALL/SOFTBALL

Warm up for at least 10 minutes. See pages 105–12 for suggestions.

EXERCISE	SETS	REP/TIME	REST
Sword Fighter p. 53	2–3	8–12	30–60 sec
Forearm Flexion & Extension p. 67	2–3	8–12	30–60 sec
Gas Pedal p. 70	2–3	8–12	30–60 sec
Reverse Curl p. 66	2–3	8–12	30–60 sec
Attachment Torso Rotation p. 95	2–3	8–12	30–60 sec
Squat p. 72	2–3	8–12	30–60 sec
Squat Shuffle p. 73	2–3	8–12	30–60 sec
Side Step p. 75	2–3	8–12	30–60 sec
Leg Curl p. 76	2–3	8–12	30–60 sec
Reverse Wood Chop p. 81	2–3	8–12	30–60 sec
Rotator Cuff—Internal Rotation p. 86	2–3	8–12	30–60 sec
Rotator Cuff—External Rotation p. 87	2–3	8–12	30–60 sec

This explosive sport requires muscular endurance, explosive speed and jumping power. Train to play weeks in advance of your season to avoid injuries. The following is a general conditioning program.

BASKETBALL

Warm up for at least 10 minutes. See pages 105–12 for suggestions.

EXERCISE	SETS	REP/TIME	REST
Frontal Raise p. 50	2–3	10–15	15–30 sec
Lateral Raise p. 51	2–3	10–15	15–30 sec
Shoulder Press p. 52	2–3	10–15	15–30 sec
Horizontal Triceps Extension p. 60	2–3	10–15	15–30 sec
Gas Pedal p. 70	2–3	10–15	15–30 sec
Squat p. 72	2–3	10–15	15–30 sec
Squat Shuffle p. 73	2–3	10–15	15–30 sec
Forward Lunge p. 74	2–3	10–15	15–30 sec
Side Step p. 75	2–3	10–15	15–30 sec
Leg Curl p. 76	2–3	10–15	15–30 sec
Attachment Lat Pull-Down p. 89	2–3	10–15	15–30 sec
Attachment Chest Flye p. 90	2–3	10–15	15–30 sec
Attachment Leg Abduction p. 91	2–3	10–15	15–30 sec
Attachment Leg Adduction p. 92	2–3	10–15	15–30 sec
Attachment Hip Extension p. 94	2–3	10–15	15–30 sec
Attachment Torso Rotation p. 95	2–3	10–15	15–30 sec
Chair Dip p. 61	2–3	10–15	15–30 sec

Biking/Cycling

Biking can range from a casual cruise to a century ride. Most people would assume that biking is a lower-body activity, but think of your posture. While biking does primarily engage the lower body, requiring muscular endurance and strength of the legs, your body is rounded over the handlebars, with much of your weight resting on your wrists and hands or shoulders. Often the lower back hurts after a long ride, thus a cyclist needs a solid core and enough strength to support the upper body and head.

A fitness program for cycling should condition all the muscles of the leg in addition to correcting the muscles of the body that are fostering poor posture. The bottom line is to increase the strength and endurance of the lower extremities by performing higher reps, as well as to condition the upper body to counteract any muscular imbalances caused by cycling. It's assumed that, if you're a regular rider, your lower body is in good shape so design a program that addresses other areas. Many of the exercises listed here can be done either standing or seated depending upon your tolerance.

BIKING/CYCLING

Warm up for at least 10 minutes. See pages 105–12 for suggestions.

EXERCISE	SETS	REP/TIME	REST
Horizontal Chest Press p. 48	2–3	8–15	15–30 sec
Shoulder Press p. 52	2–3	8–15	15–30 sec
Archery Pull p. 58	2–3	8–15	15–30 sec
Forearm Flexion & Extension p. 67	2–3	8–15	15–30 sec
Wrist Fold p. 68	2–3	8–15	15–30 sec
Racehorse p. 69	2–3	8–15	15–30 sec
Shrug p. 64	2–3	8–15	15–30 sec
Downward Sword Fighter p. 54	2–3	8–15	15–30 sec
Forward Lunge p. 74	2–3	8–15	15–30 sec
Attachment Long Row p. 88	2–3	8–15	15–30 sec
Attachment Lat Pull-Down p. 89	2–3	8–15	15–30 sec
Side Bend p. 82	2–3	8–15	15–30 sec
Hip Extension p. 78	2–3	8–15	15–30 sec
Half Sit-Up p. 80	2–3	8–15	15–30 sec
Pelvic Lift p. 84	2–3	8–15	15–30 sec
Attachment Leg Curl p. 93	2–3	8–15	15–30 sec
* Ball & Band Upright Flye p. 98	2–3	8–15	15–30 sec
* Ball & Band Bench Press p. 97	2–3	8–15	15–30 sec

* for advanced level only

Bowling

Many people don't think of bowling as a sport, yet it can be very hard on the lower back, hips and shoulders. Bowling is a one-sided activity that requires you to throw a heavy ball with significant force to knock over the pins. This can cause muscular imbalances, which can lead to injury. Resistance training can help to correct many of these issues by strengthening the total body as well as improving flexibility.

Since bowling is an activity that requires strength and power, you should work toward improving both. Therefore, once you establish a baseline of muscular strength and endurance, start focusing on doing moves more quickly. However, keep in mind that explosive moves put you at higher risk for injury, so train smart, not hard.

BOWLING

Warm up for at least 10 minutes. See pages 105–12 for suggestions.

EXERCISE	SETS	REP/TIME	REST
Pull-Down p. 45	2	8–10	30–45 sec
Reverse Flye p. 47	2	8–10	30–45 sec
Long Row p. 55	2	8–10	30–45 sec
Bike Pump p. 57	2	8–10	30–45 sec
Archery Pull p. 58	2	8–10	30–45 sec
Forearm Flexion & Extension p. 67	2–3	8–15	15–30 sec
Reverse Curl p. 66	2	8–10	30–45 sec
Racehorse p. 69	2	8–10	30–45 sec
Leg Press p. 71	2	8–10	30–45 sec
Chair Sit-Up p. 79	2	8–10	30–45 sec
Shrug p. 64	2	8–10	30–45 sec
Squat p. 72	2	8–10	30–45 sec
Reverse Wood Chop p. 81	2	8–10	30–45 sec
Side Bend p. 82	2	8–10	30–45 sec
Pelvic Lift p. 84	2	8–10	30–45 sec

Golf

Most people compete at golf, either against others or themselves. Golf is a tough game on the body, requiring twisting of the knees and lower back. This asymmetrical sport, with moves repeated sometimes up to ninety times, presents a whole set of problems. Ironically, the worse you are at the game, the harder it is on your body because you take more swings—with biomechanically incorrect form.

A golfer does not require big muscles or a lot of strength, but the game requires controlled power. Therefore, your exercise program should try to replicate the moves and the speed used on the course. For your health, a sound fitness program should also be aimed at undoing the unilateral movement, so work all the muscles of the body and keep the body fluid. After you develop a baseline of strength, increase your power by doing the moves more quickly. However, be careful—ballistic moves can cause injuries. This program offers general conditioning that focuses on leg strength and back protection.

GOLF

Warm up for at least 10 minutes. See pages 105–12 for suggestions.

EXERCISE	SETS	REP/TIME	REST
Pull-Down p. 45	2	8–10	30–45 sec
Reverse Flye p. 47	2	8–10	30–45 sec
Long Row p. 55	2	8–10	30–45 sec
Flye p. 46	2	8–10	30–45 sec
Lateral Raise p. 51	2	8–10	30–45 sec
Lawnmower Pull p. 62	2–3	8–15	15–30 sec
Forearm Flexion & Extension p. 67	2–3	8–15	15–30 sec
Reverse Curl p. 66	2	8–10	30–45 sec
Wrist Fold p. 68	2	8–10	30–45 sec
Racehorse p. 69	2	8–10	30–45 sec
Gas Pedal p. 70	2	8–10	30–45 sec
Chair Sit-Up p. 79	2	8–10	30–45 sec
Leg Press p. 71	2	8–10	30–45 sec
Upright Row p. 56	2	8–10	30–45 sec
Downward Sword Fighter p. 54	2	8–10	30–45 sec
Squat p. 72	2	8–10	30–45 sec
Forward Lunge p. 74	2	8–10	30–45 sec
Reverse Wood Chop p. 81	2	8–10	30–45 sec
Side Bend p. 82	2	8–10	30–45 sec
* Attachment Lat Pull-Down p. 89	2	8–10	30–45 sec
* Attachment Torso Rotation p. 95	2	8–10	30–45 sec

* for advanced level only

Walking and jogging are excellent aerobic activities that, unfortunately, stress the lower limbs by placing three to five times your body weight on your knees. However, the muscles of the torso are engaged as well, so when designing your routine, place most of your focus on upper-body conditioning and stretching the muscles of the lower body and back. Focus on muscular endurance more than strength and power.

A strength program for a walker/jogger will aim for higher reps with lighter load. This general conditioning program focuses on arm strength and back protection.

JOGGING/WALKING/HIKING

Warm up for at least 10 minutes. See pages 105–12 for suggestions.

EXERCISE	SETS	REP/TIME	REST
Pull-Down *p. 45*	2	8–12	20–30 sec
Reverse Flye *p. 47*	2	8–12	20–30 sec
Horizontal Chest Press *p. 48*	2	8–12	20–30 sec
Flye *p. 46*	2	8–12	20–30 sec
Frontal Raise *p. 50*	2	8–12	20–30 sec
Shoulder Press *p. 52*	2	8–12	20–30 sec
Archery Pull *p. 58*	2	8–12	20–30 sec
Biceps Curl *p. 65*	2	8–12	20–30 sec
Reverse Curl *p. 66*	2	8–12	20–30 sec
Triceps Extension *p. 59*	2	8–12	20–30 sec
Chair Sit-Up *p. 79*	2	8–12	20–30 sec
* Attachment Lat Pull-Down *p. 89*	2	8–12	20–30 sec
* Attachment Torso Rotation *p. 95*	2	8–12	20–30 sec

* for advanced level only

Skiing

Skiing can be an explosive sport that asks you to perform hard for short spurts, stand around for a while in line and then exert full force again. You also have to contend with the cold and high altitudes. Skiing, whether cross-country or downhill, is a total-body sport that requires good lower-body strength and endurance. Unfortunately, it can be hard on shoulders and knees. This total-body workout addresses muscular power and endurance.

SKIING

Warm up for at least 10 minutes. See pages 105–12 for suggestions.

EXERCISE	SETS	REP/TIME	REST
Frontal Raise p. 50	2–3	8–15	30–45 sec
Lateral Raise p. 51	2–3	8–15	30–45 sec
Shoulder Press p. 52	2–3	8–15	30–45 sec
Triceps Extension p. 59	2–3	8–15	30–45 sec
Forearm Flexion & Extension p. 67	2–3	8–15	15–30 sec
Biceps Curl p. 65	2–3	8–15	30–45 sec
Gas Pedal p. 70	2–3	8–15	30–45 sec
Squat p. 72	2–3	8–15	30–45 sec
Squat Shuffle p. 73	2–3	8–15	30–45 sec
Forward Lunge p. 74	2–3	8–15	30–45 sec
Leg Curl p. 76	2–3	8–15	30–45 sec
Hip Extension p. 78	2–3	8–15	30–45 sec
Attachment Torso Rotation p. 95	2–3	8–15	30–45 sec
Push-Up p. 85	2–3	8–15	30–45 sec
Ball & Band Bench Press p. 97	2–3	8–15	30–45 sec

Water exercise is gentle on the body and everybody should do it, but swimming is not as kind. In fact, swimming can be hard on the shoulders and even the neck and lower back if your form is faulty. Another problem arises if you don't vary your strokes—all the muscles on the front of your body get worked (and consequently get tight) while your upper back becomes hunched.

Swimming also doesn't do much for bone strengthening. This is why a compressive strength-training program is needed. The following routine attempts to address the above-mentioned issues. If you're doing a great deal of swimming, be mindful of your shoulders as you may be overtraining. You may wish to focus on working your legs and torso if your shoulders need a rest. Another consideration is to focus on corrective exercises listed such as Downward Sword Fighter, Rotator Cuff—External Rotation and Rotator Cuff—Internal Rotation.

SWIMMING

Warm up for at least 10 minutes. See pages 105–12 for suggestions.

EXERCISE	SETS	REP/TIME	REST
Reverse Flye *p. 47*	3	8–15	20–30 sec
Long Row *p. 55*	3	8–15	20–30 sec
Sword Fighter *p. 53*	3	8–15	20–30 sec
Archery Pull *p. 58*	3	8–15	20–30 sec
Downward Sword Fighter *p. 54*	3	8–15	20–30 sec
Rotator Cuff—Internal Rotation *p. 86*	3	8–15	20–30 sec
Rotator Cuff—External Rotation *p. 87*	3	8–15	20–30 sec
Half Sit-Up *p. 80*	3	8–15	20–30 sec
Pelvic Lift *p. 84*	3	8–15	20–30 sec
Ball & Band Bench Press *p. 97*	3	8–15	20–30 sec
Ball & Band Reclining Flye *p. 99*	3	8–15	20–30 sec

Tennis

Tennis is a fun activity that can be played at various levels well into old age. However, tennis does take a toll on joints such as the knees, hips, lower back and shoulders. The following program should give you enough strength to continue playing for years to come. Since tennis is an explosive sport that requires bursts of speed and power, once you establish a baseline of muscular strength and endurance, your program should start focusing on developing power by doing moves more quickly. However, keep in mind that explosive moves put you at more risk for injury, so train smart, not hard.

TENNIS

Warm up for at least 10 minutes. See pages 105–12 for suggestions.

EXERCISE	SETS	REP/TIME	REST
Reverse Flye p. 47	2–3	8–12	20–30 sec
Standing Frontal Raise p. 50	2–3	8–12	20–30 sec
Sword Fighter p. 53	2–3	8–12	20–30 sec
Forearm Flexion & Extension p. 67	2–3	8–15	15–30 sec
Wrist Fold p. 68	2–3	8–12	20–30 sec
Racehorse p. 69	2–3	8–12	20–30 sec
Gas Pedal p. 70	2–3	8–12	20–30 sec
Squat Shuffle p. 73	2–3	8–12	20–30 sec
Forward Lunge p. 74	2–3	8–12	20–30 sec
Reverse Wood Chop p. 81	2–3	8–12	20–30 sec
Side Bend p. 82	2–3	8–12	20–30 sec
Crescent Moon p. 83	2–3	8–12	20–30 sec
Rotator Cuff—Internal p. 86	2–3	8–12	20–30 sec
Rotator Cuff—External p. 87	2–3	8–12	20–30 sec
Attachment Leg Abduction p. 91	2–3	8–12	20–30 sec
Attachment Leg Adduction p. 92	2–3	8–12	20–30 sec
Attachment Hip Extension p. 94	2–3	8–12	20–30 sec
Attachment Torso Rotation p. 95	2–3	8–12	20–30 sec
Half Sit-Up p. 80	2–3	8–12	20–30 sec
Pelvic Lift p. 84	2–3	8–12	20–30 sec
Ball & Band Upright Flye p. 98	2–3	8–12	20–30 sec

Stiffness and chronic pain are common characteristics of arthritis, and the phrase "use it or lose it" really applies here: If you don't move that joint, it will become stiffer and weaker. Unfortunately, many people with arthritis are afraid to exercise in fear that they'll make the condition worse. As the person with arthritis starts to do less, the muscles weaken, which in turn puts more load and strain on an already-compromised joint. However, recent research supports that having arthritis is not an excuse not to exercise. Stronger joints serve as a better support system for compromised knees, hips and more. The trick is to find the correct dose of exercise to obtain the correct response. Keep in mind that, as with any chronic condition, you'll have periods of exacerbation. On those days it's OK to only do the easy exercises.

Of course, you should always consult with your doctor or therapist before starting a routine, but here are some sound recommendations when exercising with arthritis:

- Always follow medical advice.
- Remember the two-hour rule: If you hurt more two hours post-exercise than when you started, do less next time.

ARTHRITIS

Warm up for at least 10 minutes. See pages 105–12 for suggestions.

EXERCISE	SETS	REP/TIME	REST
Pull-Down p. 45	1	6–12	30–45 sec
Horizontal Chest Press p. 48	1	6–12	30–45 sec
Reverse Flye p. 47	1	6–12	30–45 sec
Frontal Raise p. 50	1	6–12	30–45 sec
Horizontal Triceps Extension p. 60	1	6–12	30–45 sec
Biceps Curl p. 65	1	6–12	30–45 sec
Gas Pedal p. 70	1	6–12	30–45 sec
Leg Press p. 71	1	6–12	30–45 sec

- On days when you don't feel like exercising, do 5 minutes and then re-assess your mood.
- Never overexercise.
- Don't mask pain with medication.
- Never exercise a swollen or "hot" joint.
- Warm up completely or maybe even take a warm shower before you start with gentle exercises; ice problematic joints if needed after a session.
- Keep movements within the pain-free range of motion.
- Avoid extreme flexion and extension.

Gentle stretching can be useful, as long as you stretch the parts you're using. A mild-to-moderate strength-training routine can go a long way in preventing further atrophy of the muscles that support the joint. Often strong muscles can replace weak joints.

No matter what type of arthritis you have, it's critical that you don't cause any further harm to the joint. Here's a basic program that can be increased as you improve. If any exercise hurts, back off and consult your doctor. As you progress, consider checking in with your medical professional as to which additional exercises would work well for you.

Back Pain

Lower back pain is caused by a variety of issues, including weak abdominal muscles, tight hamstrings and quadriceps, improper body mechanics, poor posture, overuse and arthritis. A healthy back program includes exercises that strengthen the abdominals and lower back muscles and stretch the hamstrings and lower back muscles. Learning and maintaining neutral spine is also very important.

Core training supports the spine by strengthening the muscles that surround the spine and torso, commonly called the "core." It's much like building your own internal back brace. Think of your body as a sunflower: Develop a solid stem to hold the flower tall.

A sound resistance training program coupled with a gentle aerobic exercise routine, a daily flexibility program and staying at an ideal weight to take the load of the joints will help facilitate positive outcomes. However, be cautious about overdoing back training or performing questionable movements that can easily bring on another bout of back pain. If any exercise hurts, back off and consult your doctor.

Keep in mind these guidelines when exercising with lower back pain:

BACK PAIN

Warm up for at least 10 minutes. See pages 105–12 for suggestions.

EXERCISE	SETS	REP/TIME	REST
Pull-Down p. 45	1	8–12	30–45 sec
Horizontal Chest Press p. 48	1	8–12	30–45 sec
Shoulder Press p. 52	1	8–12	30–45 sec
Horizontal Triceps Extension p. 60	1	8–12	30–45 sec
Biceps Curl p. 65	1	8–12	30–45 sec
Attachment Lat Pull-Down p. 89	1	8–12	30–45 sec

- Always follow medical advice.
- Remember the two-hour rule: If you hurt more two hours post-exercise than when you started, do less next time.
- On days when you don't feel like exercising, do 5 minutes and then re-assess your mood.
- Never overexercise.
- Don't mask pain with medication.
- Never exercise a swollen or "hot" joint.
- Warm up completely or maybe even take a warm shower before you start with gentle exercises; ice problematic joints if needed after a session.
- Keep movements within the pain-free range of motion.
- Avoid extreme flexion and extension.
- If you notice an increase in pain and/or numbness in your legs or feet, stop and see your health professional.
- Avoid overhead lifts and bending-over moves that place load on your spine.

Often called the workhorse of the body, the hip joint is designed to support the load of your body and plays a significant role in many activities of daily living, from climbing stairs to walking. Unfortunately, some people overuse them with their jobs or in the weight room with heavy lifts. Years of being overweight can also cause good hips to go bad. If you've had a hip replacement, consult your health professional for specific exercises. The focus of this program is mobility and stability of the hip region. If you have severe hip issues, always consult a health professional first. This program is designed to be a preventive program and in some cases a corrective routine.

Keep in mind these guidelines when exercising with hip issues:

- Avoid flexion past 90 degrees (allowing your knee to get too close to your chest).
- Avoid crossing the midline of your body (when you swing your leg in front or behind the other leg).
- Keep hip, knee and ankle in alignment when doing leg presses and squats.
- Avoid full squats.

HIP ISSUES

Warm up for at least 10 minutes. See pages 105–12 for suggestions.

EXERCISE	SETS	REP/TIME	REST
Gas Pedal p. 70	1–2	8–12	30–45 sec
Leg Press p. 71	1–2	8–12	30–45 sec
Squat p. 72	1–2	8–12	30–45 sec
* Squat Shuffle p. 73	1–2	8–12	30–45 sec
* Forward Lunge p. 74	1–2	8–12	30–45 sec
* Side Step p. 75	1–2	8–12	30–45 sec
Leg Curl p. 76	1–2	8–12	30–45 sec
Side Bend p. 82	1–2	8–12	30–45 sec
Attachment Leg Abduction p. 91	1–2	8–12	30–45 sec
Attachment Leg Adduction p. 92	1–2	8–12	30–45 sec
Attachment Hip Extension p. 94	1–2	8–12	30–45 sec

* perform with caution

Knee Issues

Your knee is an engineering marvel but it can still break down if used incorrectly. The knees are designed to straighten and bend; any other movement puts them at some level of risk. Chronic knee problems can be the result of poor anatomical design. If you're bowlegged or knock-kneed, you're at a mechanical disadvantage that can set you up for injury. Foot misalignments can also contribute to knee problems. The causes of knee problems are many and range from arthritis to torn ligaments caused from misuse and abuse. See your doctor to get a proper diagnosis and corrective suggestions.

Simple activities such as jogging or even walking can increase the load on the knee joint three to five times the person's body weight. In addition, sports injuries from soccer, football or even biking with poor form can harm your knees. To reduce knee pain, strengthen all the muscles of your quads and if appropriate lose excess body weight/fat. Strength-training exercises should not increase pain or swelling. If it's OK with your health professional, apply ice after a training session.

KNEE ISSUES

Warm up for at least 10 minutes. See pages 105–12 for suggestions.

EXERCISE	SETS	REP/TIME	REST
Squat p. 72	2–3	8–12	30–45 sec
Forward Lunge p. 74	2–3	8–12	30–45 sec
Leg Curl p. 76	2–3	8–12	30–45 sec
Pelvic Lift p. 84	2–3	8–12	30–45 sec

The following guidelines may serve useful:

- Always point the knees and toes in the same direction.
- Avoid any movements that make your knees rotate or twist, and never twist your body while your feet are planted on the floor.
- Never straighten your knee so far that it overly straightens the leg.
- Avoid thigh stretches that cause your knees to bend too much. Forcing your knee to bend too far overstretches the knee ligaments and can make the joint unstable.
- Avoid deep knee bends/full squats, and make sure you don't squat any lower than the point at which your thighs are parallel to the floor.
- Always remember: Keep your knees "soft" (that is, slightly bent) when stretching.
- Don't allow the knee to extend past the toes.
- Never go past your safe range of motion.
- If you're told to wear a brace when exercising, be sure to follow all recommendations.
- Use caution when doing leg-extension exercises.
- Aim to do two to three sets of 8–12 reps, but listen to your body so that you don't exacerbate any issues.

Osteoporosis is a silent disease; the first sign of it is often a fracture. A quick turn can cause the hip joint to snap; a simple fall can result in a fracture of the wrist or, even worse, a broken hip. This section is included for all ages. Both men and women need to realize that osteoporosis is a disease that starts in childhood but manifests itself in old age. Too often when a diagnosis of osteoporosis is given, it's too late to do much other than live with the effects of stooped posture and chronic back pain. The medical community can offer medications, but prevention is the best treatment.

Fortunately, osteoporosis is not inevitable. It's never too late to be pro-active. With the help of your physician, changes to your lifestyle along with a sensible proper weight-bearing exercise program can make good things happen to your bones because your bones are living structures that are re-modeling themselves every day. Research has shown that when muscles get stronger, the bones will get stronger too. Also, when you get stronger hopefully you'll be strong enough to catch your balance and not fall (falls are a major reason

OSTEOPOROSIS

Warm up for at least 10 minutes. Start easily and lightly and progress carefully. See pages 105–12 for suggestions.

EXERCISE	SETS	REP/TIME	REST
Reverse Flye *p. 47*	1–2	8–15	30–45 sec
Horizontal Chest Press *p. 48*	1–2	8–15	30–45 sec
Archery Pull *p. 58*	1–2	8–15	30–45 sec
Horizontal Triceps Extension *p. 60*	1–2	8–15	30–45 sec
Leg Press *p. 71*	1–2	8–15	30–45 sec
Forward Lunge *p. 74*	1–2	8–15	30–45 sec

why older people end up in the hospital and can die as a result of injuries sustained). If you only have osteopenia (early-stage osteoporosis), beginning strength training right now may prevent you from ever developing full-blown osteoporosis. It's never too early to start—the bones you build today are the bones that will support you tomorrow.

Benefits of strength-training exercises if you have osteoporosis:
- Improved balance and gait to prevent falling
- Improved flexibility so you have a more fluid gait to prevent falling
- Reversed muscle atrophy, which can prevent falls
- Good stresses on bones that stimulate thickening of the bones and improve their density

Here are some guidelines to keep in mind when training with resistance bands:
- Be careful when bending forward or twisting.
- Use caution when lifting overhead.
- Always stay mindful of proper posture and body mechanics.

This basic starter program should be paired with a gentle walking program.

Shoulder Issues

The design of the shoulder is remarkable, allowing a baseball pitcher to throw a ball 90 mph or allowing a person to rock a baby to sleep. The shoulder is a ball-and-socket joint that gets its support from muscles, ligaments and tendons. The more active you are, the greater the risk of injuring your shoulder. Shoulder problems can be the result of many things, including bursitis and tendonitis, or they can arise from no known cause.

Many times the corrective exercises given to you by your health professional will be the same regardless of the cause. Often the recommendation given to people with shoulder issues is to stretch what is tight and strengthen what is weak. But it's still wise to have a medical doctor provide you with a proper diagnosis and have a physical therapist give you specific corrective exercises.

Here are some guidelines when training with a shoulder issue:

- Avoid overhead arm exercises or any moves that increase pain and/or limit your range of motion.
- Follow directions exactly when doing movements that involve the shoulder joint.

SHOULDER ISSUES			
Warm up for at least 10 minutes. See pages 105–12 for suggestions.			
EXERCISE	SETS	REP/TIME	REST
Reverse Flye p. 47	1–2	5–7	30–45 sec
Long Row p. 55	1–2	5–7	30–45 sec
Sword Fighter p. 53	1–2	5–7	30–45 sec
Archery Pull p. 58	1–2	5–7	30–45 sec
Shrug p. 64	1–2	5–7	30–45 sec
Downward Sword Fighter p. 54	1–2	5–7	30–45 sec
Rotator Cuff—Internal p. 86	1–2	5–7	30–45 sec
Rotator Cuff—External p. 87	1–2	5–7	30–45 sec
Attachment Lat Pull-Down p. 89	1–2	5–7	30–45 sec

- Strength-training exercises should not increase pain. If it's OK with your health professional, apply ice after a training session.
- Participate in shoulder and chest flexibility exercises.
- When doing frontal or lateral raises, don't go higher than your shoulders.
- Always control any movement that causes you to raise your arms above shoulder height.
- Relax your shoulders and don't shrug when you're doing arm exercises.
- Try your best to keep your shoulder blades pulled together when doing arm moves.
- If your shoulders are tight, don't arch your back to make up for your inflexibility.
- Stretch your chest and shoulder area regularly.

Wrist Issues

Wrist pain is becoming increasingly common with people spending so much time texting and using the computer. General exercises of the wrist and forearm could be helpful. If an exercise exacerbates your symptoms, stop immediately.

WRIST ISSUES

Warm up for at least 10 minutes. See pages 105–12 for suggestions.

EXERCISE	SETS	REP/TIME	REST
Forearm Flexion & Extension p. 67	2–3	8–15	15–30 sec
Wrist Fold p. 68	1–2	8–15	30–45 sec
Racehorse p. 69	1–2	8–15	30–45 sec

Diabetes

There are two types of diabetes mellitus: juvenile diabetes, or type 1 diabetes, and adult-onset diabetes, or type 2 diabetes. When a person has diabetes, the body does not provide enough of the hormone insulin, which helps regulate the amount of sugar in the bloodstream. Regular exercise and healthy eating habits can help a person with diabetes stabilize the condition. Having diabetes or being at risk for developing diabetes is not an excuse not to exercise but rather a reason to exercise. As with any other chronic condition, prior to starting an exercise program consult with your health professional for any special recommendations and precautions specific to you.

Here are some helpful guidelines to follow:

- Avoid activities that are stressful to your feet.
- Extended warm-up and cool-down periods are important for diabetics when transitioning from moderate exercise to rest.
- Avoid heavy, intense exercise.
- Train at a pace that allows you to hold a conversation.
- Be alert of your insulin and blood sugar levels.
- If you're injecting insulin, be mindful of where the injection is and what set of muscles you're planning to use. Discuss with your health professional about appropriate injection sites when exercising. A general tip is not to inject the area that you'll be exercising that day.
- If you have retinal issues, speak with your eye doctor before starting.

DIABETES

Warm up for at least 15 minutes. See pages 105–12 for suggestions.

EXERCISE	SETS	REP/TIME	REST
Seated Horizontal Chest Press p. 48	1–2	8–15	30–45 sec
Archery Pull p. 58	1–2	8–15	30–45 sec
Gas Pedal p. 70	1–2	8–15	30–45 sec
Leg Press p. 71	1–2	8–15	30–45 sec
Standing Frontal Raise p. 50	1–2	8–15	30–45 sec
Shrug p. 64	1–2	8–15	30–45 sec
Biceps Curl p. 65	1–2	8–15	30–45 sec
Triceps Extension p. 59	1–2	8–15	30–45 sec

Blood pressure fluctuates from moment to moment and is affected by everything from stress and environmental stimulation to physical exertion. High blood pressure is a major risk factor in developing a stroke, heart disease and several other health issues. Numerous studies have shown that aerobic exercise has a positive influence on lowering blood pressure. Use caution if you choose to strength train as heavy strength training can elevate your blood pressure to dangerous levels. It's wise to ask your doctor if resistance training is OK for you before starting.

Here are some guidelines for a safe workout:

- Emphasize muscular endurance over strength and power. The goal should be to do a higher number of reps with a lighter load.
- If your blood pressure is above 160/90, check with your doctor before resistance training.
- Be careful of overhead moves.
- Always make time to adequately warm up and cool down. People with vascular issues such as high or low blood pressure can get into trouble if they start out too hard and stop exercising abruptly. Be alert that blood pressure medications can cause sudden drops in blood pressure with postural moves such as getting up too quickly.
- Don't hold your breath while training.
- Ask your doctor what influence your medication has on exercise.
- If you can't whistle while you're exercising, you're working too hard.

HIGH BLOOD PRESSURE

Warm up for at least 10 minutes. See pages 105–12 for suggestions. For this general workout, be sure to use a light band.

EXERCISE	SETS	REP/TIME	REST
Seated Reverse Flye p. 47	1–2	8–15	30–45 sec
Seated Horizontal Chest Press p. 48	1–2	8–15	30–45 sec
Seated Archery Pull p. 58	1–2	8–15	30–45 sec
Gas Pedal p. 70	1–2	8–15	30–45 sec
Leg Press p. 71	1–2	8–15	30–45 sec

Breathing Conditions

Chronic obstructive pulmonary disease (COPD) is a progressive disorder of the lungs characterized by the destruction of the alveoli, retention of mucus secretions and so on. Common conditions grouped under this heading include bronchitis, asthma, emphysema and sometime allergies—all of which make breathing difficult. It's common to see individuals who have COPD not engage in much activity. However, research shows that a slow, progressive overall fitness program often leads to better aerobic fitness, which in turn leads to a better quality of life.

A comprehensive COPD program should improve ventilation, improve strength and endurance of respiratory muscles, maintain and improve chest and back mobility, improve leg strength to make activities of daily living easier and teach effective breathing patterns. It's highly recommended that your program be tailored to your particular health issues by a health professional.

Here are tips for a comfortable exercise session:

- Include several rest breaks during your gentle strength-training program.
- Start very, very slowly. Avoid getting out of breath.

BREATHING CONDITIONS

Warm up for at least 10 minutes. See pages 105–12 for suggestions.

EXERCISE	SETS	REP/TIME	REST
Long Row *p. 55*	1	8–15	30–45 sec
Seated Shoulder Press *p. 52*	1	8–15	30–45 sec
Biceps Curl *p. 65*	1	8–15	30–45 sec
Seated Triceps Extension *p. 59*	1	8–15	30–45 sec
Squat *p. 72*	1	8–15	30–45 sec
Forward Lunge *p. 74*	1	8–15	30–45 sec

- Never overextend yourself. It's better to do 1–2 minutes of exercise, rest and then repeat your bout of exercise when ready. Aim to work up to 10–15 minutes of non-stop exercise if possible.
- Learn how to do "pursed-lip breathing" from your health care provider and follow their recommendations. If you use an inhaler, consult your doctor about exercising and the use of the device.
- Ask your physician if you should monitor your O_2 levels when exercising.

Sarcopenia is age-related muscle loss, often related to doing less as we age. Muscles are the furnaces that rev up our metabolism. All too often as we age we find that doing simple activities of daily living fatigues us. The intervention is a daily dose of resistance band training. Research has shown that even people in their 80s and 90s can improve in strength. The following program is a great place to start. It's very easy and should only take 5 minutes to complete.

SARCOPENIA

Warm up for at least 10 minutes. See pages 105–12 for suggestions.

EXERCISE	SETS	REP/TIME	REST
Pull-Down p. 45	1	8–15	30–45 sec
Horizontal Chest Press p. 48	1	8–15	30–45 sec
Horizontal Triceps Extension p. 60	1	8–15	30–45 sec
Gas Pedal p. 70	1	8–15	30–45 sec
Leg Press p. 71	1	8–15	30–45 sec

PART 3

the

exercises

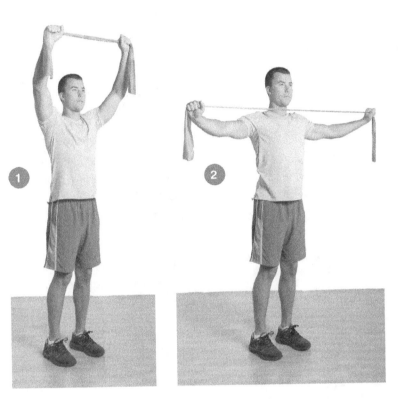

1 Sit or stand with proper posture and grasp the band with both hands at a location wide enough to provide the desired resistance. Take your arms overhead but slightly angled forward.

2 Keeping your wrists neutral (don't bend them) and your head and upper back in proper posture, slowly pull both ends of the band downward until your hands are at shoulder height. Pause.

Slowly return to start position.

SINGLE-ARM VARIATION:
This can also be done one arm at a time. Alternate between left and right arms.

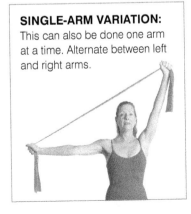

1 Sit or stand with proper posture and place the band behind your mid-upper back. Grasp the band in each hand in front of your shoulders and open your arms out to the sides.

2 Keeping your wrists neutral (don't bend them) and your head and upper back in proper posture, slowly bring your hands toward each other in front of your shoulders.

Keeping tension in your arms, slowly return to start position.

INCLINE VARIATION:
Extend the arms upward at a 45-degree angle before taking them out to the sides.

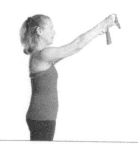

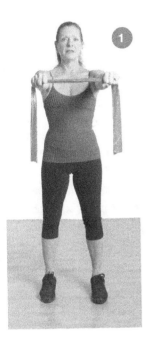

1 Sit or stand with proper posture and grasp the band with both hands in front of your chest. Extend your arms straight out in front of you. Adjust your grip until you have the desired resistance.

2 Keeping your arms parallel to the floor, your wrists neutral (don't bend them) and your head and upper back in proper posture, slowly open your arms out to the sides.

Slowly return to start position.

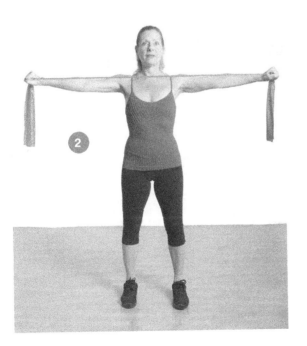

horizontal chest press

1 Sit or stand with proper posture and place the band behind your mid-upper back. Grasp the band in each hand at a point of adequate resistance in front of your shoulders.

2 Keeping your wrists neutral (don't bend them) and your head and upper back in proper posture, slowly press both ends of the band forward. Pause when your arms are extended in front of you.

Slowly return to start position.

SINGLE-ARM VARIATION:
This can also be done one arm at a time. Alternate between left and right arms.

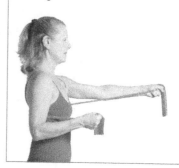

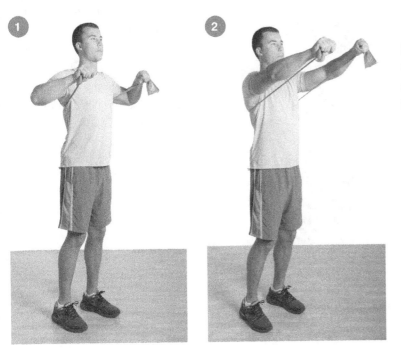

1 Sit or stand with proper posture and place the band behind your mid-upper back. Grasp the band in each hand at a point of adequate resistance in front of your shoulders.

2 Keeping your wrists neutral (don't bend them) and your head and upper back in proper posture, slowly press both ends of the band forward and upward at a 45-degree angle. Pause when your arms are extended in front of you.

Slowly return to start position.

1 Sit or stand on the middle of the band with the band in each hand. Place your arms alongside your body with your palms facing your thighs. Adjust your grip on the band until it provides the desired resistance.

2 Keeping your arms straight, slowly raise your arms forward no higher than shoulder height.

Slowly return to start position.

SINGLE-ARM VARIATION: This can also be done one arm at a time. Alternate between left and right arms.

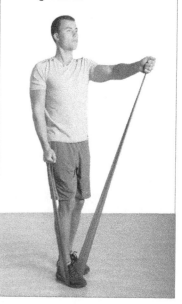

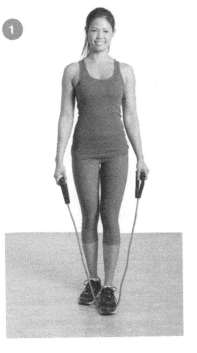

1 Sit or stand on the middle of the band with the band in each hand. Place your arms alongside your body with your palms facing your body. Adjust your grip on the band until it provides the desired resistance.

2 Keeping your arms straight, slowly raise your arms to the sides no higher than shoulder height.

Slowly return to start position.

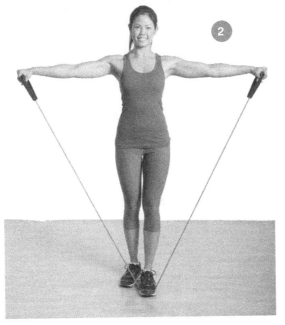

SINGLE-ARM VARIATION: This can also be done one arm at a time. Alternate between left and right arms.

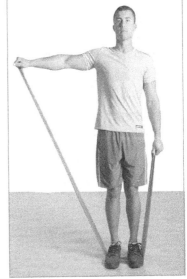

①

②

This can be performed while sitting in a chair or standing.

Caution: Do not perform this exercise if you have a history of shoulder concerns.

1 Sit or stand with proper posture and place the band behind your mid-upper back and under your armpits. Grasp the band in each hand in front of your shoulders at a location that provides adequate resistance.

2 Keeping your wrists neutral (don't bend them) and your head and upper back in proper posture, slowly press both ends of the band up toward the ceiling. Pause when your arms are extended.

Slowly return to start position.

SINGLE-ARM VARIATION:
This can also be done one arm at a time. Alternate between left and right arms.

MODIFICATION: If you have a shoulder issue, you can press the band slightly forward to lessen the strain on the shoulder joint.

VARIATION (pictured): You can also sit or stand on the middle of the band and bring an end of the band in each hand to shoulder height.

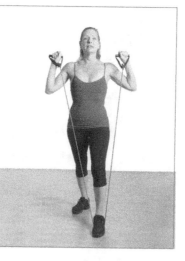

1 Sit or stand upright. Use your left hand to secure an end of the band to your left hip then grasp the band with your right hand at a location that provides your desired resistance.

2 Keeping your right arm straight, slowly pull the band diagonally across your body as if pulling out a sword from its sheath.

Slowly return to start position. Repeat, then switch sides.

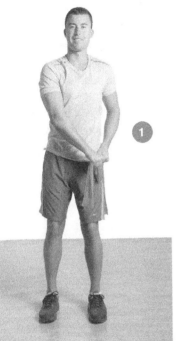

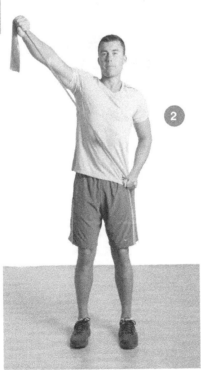

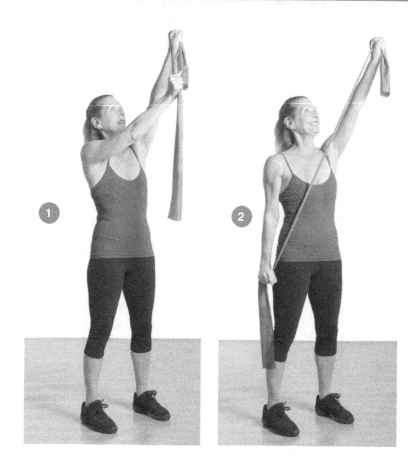

1 Sit or stand with proper posture. With your left hand, hold the end of the band slightly above your head. Grasp the band with your right hand at a location that provides adequate resistance.

2 Slowly pull your right hand down diagonally to your right hip.

Slowly return to start position. Repeat, then switch sides.

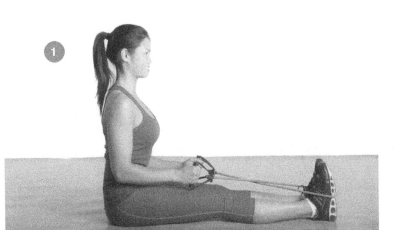

1 Sit on the floor, wrap the band around your feet and extend your legs in front of you. Grasp the band in each hand at a location that provides the desired resistance.

2 Keeping your wrists neutral (don't bend them) and your head and upper back in proper posture, slowly pull both ends of the band toward your chest. Pause when the band is near your chest.

Slowly return to start position.

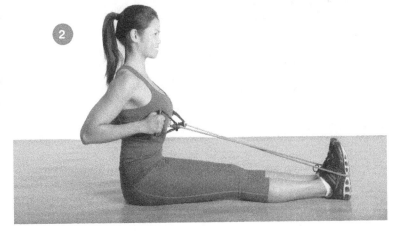

SINGLE-ARM VARIATION:
This can also be done while sitting in a chair. Extend your leg(s) forward once you've wrapped the band around your foot/feet.

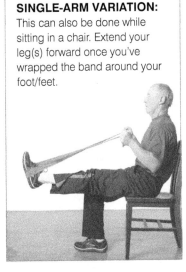

1

2

If you have a shoulder concern, be careful and start with a small range of motion and an easy band.

1 Stand in the middle of the band with an end of the band in each hand and your knees softly bent. Your hands should be in front of your hips, palms facing your body. Adjust your grip on the band until you have your desired resistance.

2 Bring the band up toward your chin, allowing your elbows to flare to the side.

Slowly return to start position.

SINGLE-ARM VARIATION:
This can also be done one arm at a time (it might be your only option if you have a short band). Alternate between left and right arms.

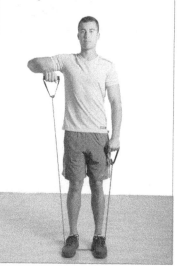

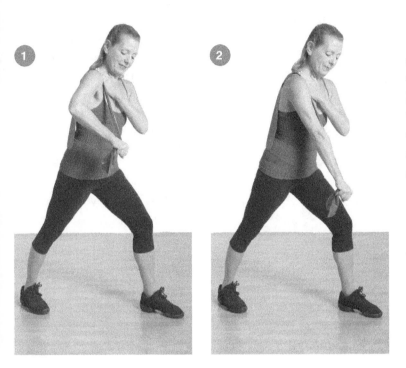

1 Stand with proper posture. Drape the band over your right shoulder and secure it in place with your left hand. With your right hand, grab the band at a location that provides ideal resistance. Once the band is in place, lean over slightly as if pushing down on a bike pump.

2 Slowly press your right arm down.

Slowly return to start position. Repeat, then switch sides.

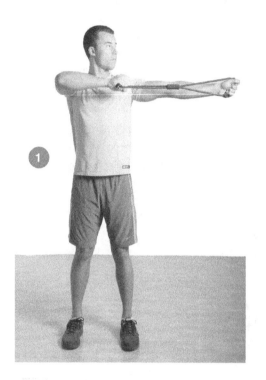

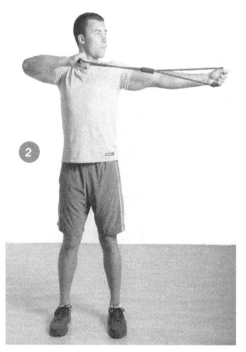

1 Sit or stand with proper posture. Hold one end of the band in your left hand and extend your left arm straight out to the side. With your right hand, grasp the band near your left elbow or shoulder at a location that provides proper resistance.

2 Pull your right arm across your chest, drawing your elbow to your right side.

Slowly return to start position. Repeat, then switch sides.

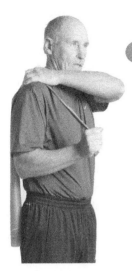

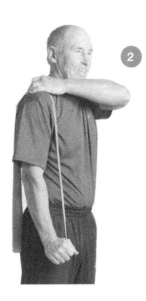

1 Stand with proper posture. Drape the band over your right shoulder and secure the band by placing your left hand on top of it. Bend your right elbow roughly 90 degrees and place it next to your ribs. With your right hand, grasp the band at a location that provides your desired resistance.

2 Without using momentum, slowly extend your right arm and hold for 1–2 seconds.

3 Slowly return your arm to a 90-degree position.

Repeat, then switch sides.

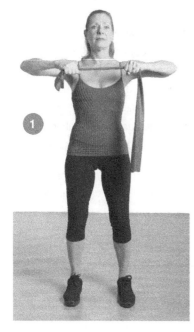

1 Sit or stand with proper posture and grasp the band with both hands approximately shoulder-width apart and at chest height. Lift your elbows out to the sides, keeping your arms parallel to the floor.

2 Keeping your right hand in place, slowly extend your left arm out to the side.

Slowly return to start position. Repeat, then switch sides.

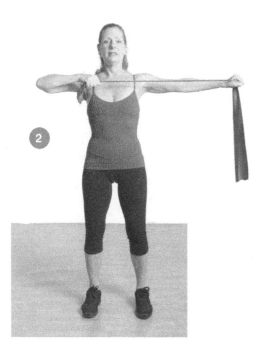

DOUBLE-ARM VARIATION: Perform the motion with both arms at the same time.

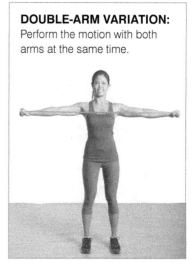

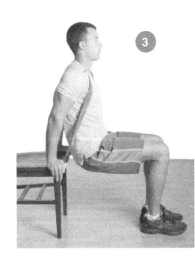

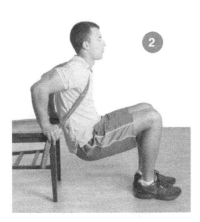

1 Sit at the edge of the chair with your feet on the floor. Place the band over your shoulders and behind your neck. With the band secure in each hand, place your palms on the seat of the chair with your fingers slightly off the seat. Slide your rear end off the chair.

2 Lower yourself down as far as is comfortable.

3 Extend your arms to raise your body.

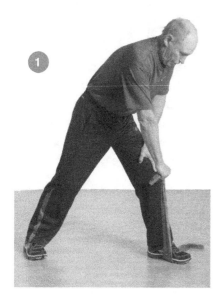

1 Step on the band with your left foot, lean over slightly as if to pull the cord on a lawnmower and then with your right hand grasp the band at a location that provides adequate resistance.

2 Pull the band up and back.

Slowly return to start position. Repeat, then switch sides.

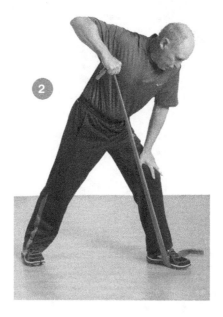

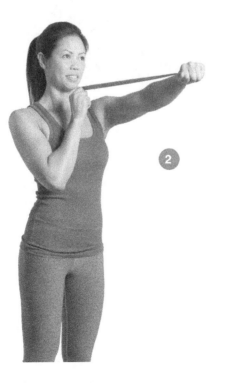

1 Sit or stand with proper posture and hold an end of the band near your mouth with your right hand. With your left hand, grasp the band at a location that provides adequate resistance.

2 Press the band forward as if sliding a trombone.

Slowly return to start position. Repeat, then switch sides.

1 Stand in the middle of the band with an end of the band in each hand and your knees softly bent. Your hands should be in front of your hips, palms facing your body. Adjust your grip on the band until you have your desired resistance.

2 Keeping your arms straight, slowly "shrug" your shoulders. Hold at the top for 1–2 seconds.

Slowly return to start position.

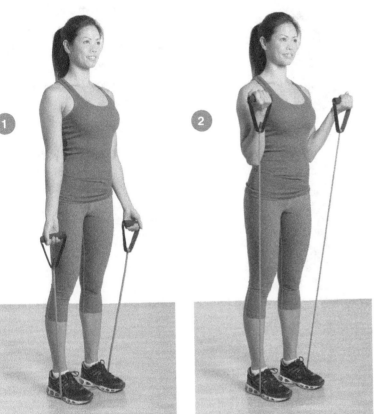

1 Stand in the middle of the band and hold an end of the band in each hand with your palms facing forward. Adjust your grip on the band until you have your desired resistance.

2 Keeping your elbows close to your ribs, bend your arms to slowly bring your palms toward your shoulders.

Slowly lower your arms.

target: biceps, forearms

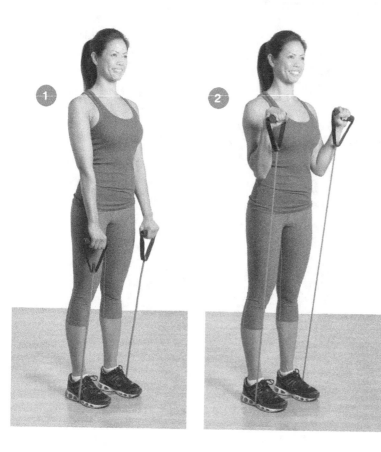

1 Stand in the middle of the band and hold an end of the band in each hand with your palms facing your body. Adjust your grip on the band until you have your desired resistance.

2 Keeping your elbows close to your ribs, bend your arms to slowly bring your knuckles toward your shoulders.

Slowly lower your arms.

SINGLE-ARM VARIATION: This can also be done with one arm.

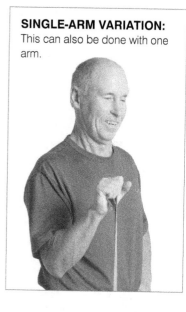

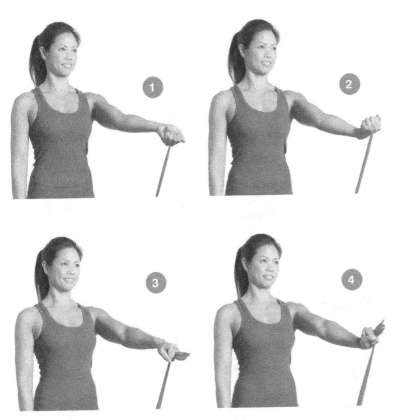

This can be performed while sitting in a chair or standing. To reduce stress on your wrist, allow the band to run between your ring and middle fingers.

1 Grasp one end of the band in your left hand and step securely on the band with your left foot at a location that provides adequate resistance. Extend your arm straight out in front of you with your palm facing up.

2 Slowly curl (flex) your palm toward your body. Pause.

Slowly return to start position. Repeat, then switch sides.

3 Now extend your arm straight out in front of you with your palm facing down.

4 Raise the back of your hand toward your body.

Slowly return to start position. Repeat, then switch sides.

SEATED MODIFICATION: With the band in your left hand, place your left forearm on your left thigh with your palm up or down. Your forearm should stay on your thigh as you flex and relax the wrist joint.

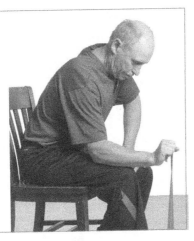

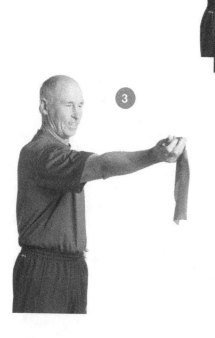

1 Sit or stand with proper posture and extend your arm while holding one end of the band.

2–3 Slowly turn your palm up, grab some band then rotate your hand and grab more band. Continue rotating your hand until the band is inside your palm. Once the band is inside your hand, squeeze it firmly ten times.

Repeat, then switch sides.

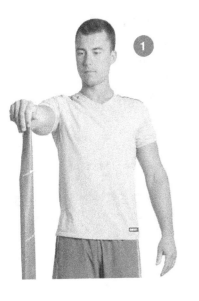

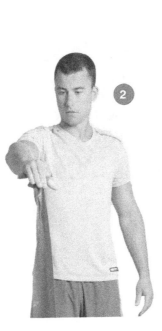

1 Sit or stand with proper posture and extend your arm while holding one end of the band.

2–3 Quickly grab some band and pull it into the palm of your hand while squeezing the band. Continue until the entire band is inside your palm. Once the band is inside your hand, squeeze it firmly ten times.

Repeat, then switch sides.

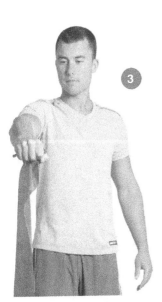

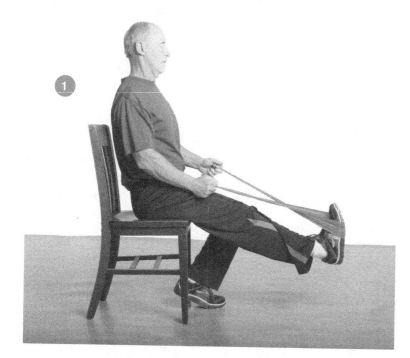

1 Sit with proper posture. Place one foot on the floor and extend the other leg straight out in front of you. Wrap the band around the ball of your foot once to keep it in place.

2 Slowly point your foot, keeping tension in the band.

Return your foot to neutral. Repeat, then switch sides.

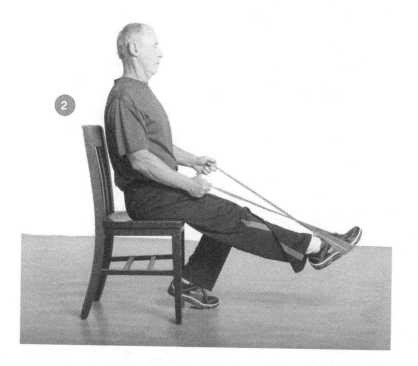

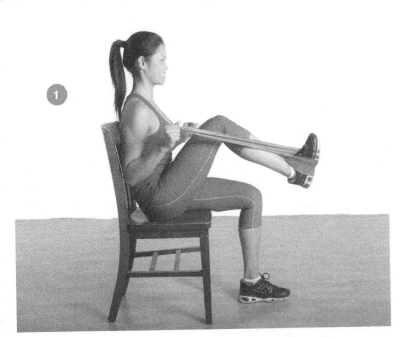

1 Sit with proper posture in the middle of a chair. Place one foot on the floor and extend the other leg straight out in front of you. Wrap the band once around the ball of the foot of the straightened leg to keep it in place. Slowly bring your knee in toward your chest.

2 Extend your leg, making sure not to lock your knee.

Return to start position. Repeat, then switch sides.

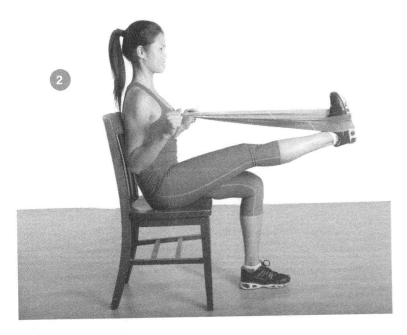

1 Stand with your feet on the center of the band. Grasp an end of the band in each hand at a place that offers your desired resistance.

2 Keeping your back in neutral position, squat down halfway, adjusting the resistance as necessary. Don't allow your knees to extend past your toes. Pause.

Return to start position.

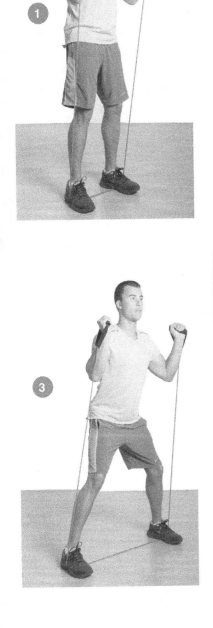

1 Stand with your feed on the center of the band. Grasp an end of the band in each hand at a place that offers your desired resistance.

2–3 Squat either a quarter- or halfway down then take several steps to the right. Do not allow your knees to extend past your toes.

Now take several steps to the left. Continue stepping to the left and right.

VARIATION: You can also wrap a tubular band around your legs at mid-thigh or tie a band around them.

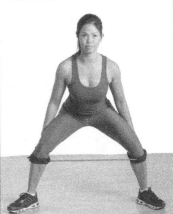

forward lunge

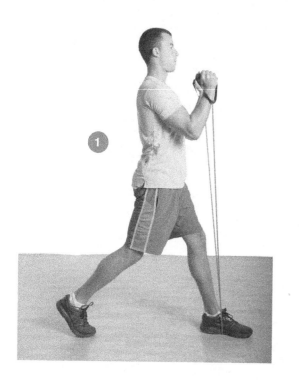

1 Stand in the middle of the band with your left foot and hold on to the band with each hand at a location that provides adequate resistance. Slide your right foot backward.

2 Attempt to lower your right knee to the floor if possible, otherwise just go as low as is comfortable. You should feel an increase in resistance in the left leg as you come upright.

Repeat, then switch sides.

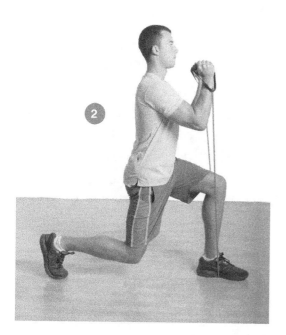

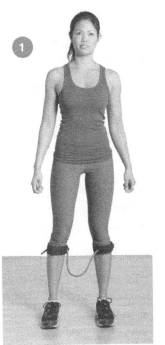

Caution: If you have hip or knee issues, proceed carefully.

1 Wrap a tubular band around your legs at mid-thigh or tie a band around both thighs.

2 Take 4 steps to the right—do not overstride—and then take 4 steps to the left.

Continue stepping to the left and right.

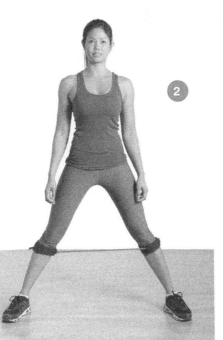

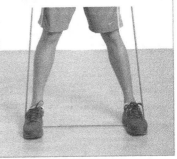

VARIATION: This can also be done while standing on the band.

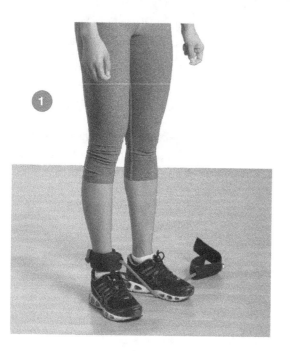

If balance is an issue, you may want to stand near a secure location for assistance.

Caution: Be careful of hamstring cramps.

1 Place a tubular band under one foot and wrap the band around the other ankle, or tie one end of the band around the ankle. Wrap the band so that it provides resistance through the full range of motion.

2 Maintaining neutral spine position, slowly curl the leg that has the band around the ankle halfway up. Control the motion in both directions—don't allow the band to determine the speed. Hold for 1–2 seconds.

Slowly lower the leg to start position. Repeat, then switch sides.

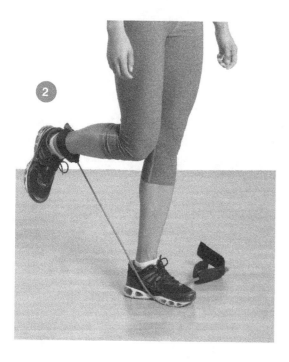

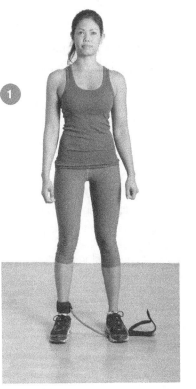

If you have balance issues, hold onto something for stability.

Caution: Avoid this exercise if you have hip problems.

1 Secure the band around each ankle, or step on the band with your left foot and wrap the other end around your right ankle. Adjust the band so that it provides resistance through the full range of motion.

2 Slowly move your right leg to the side a comfortable distance.

Slowly lower the leg to start position. Repeat, then switch sides.

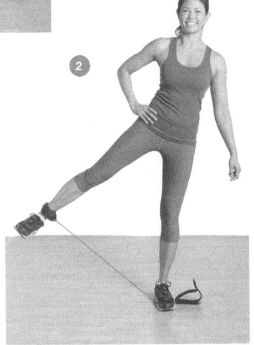

SEATED MODIFICATION: Wrap the band around your thighs and then slowly separate your knees.

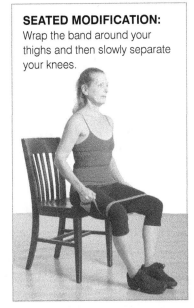

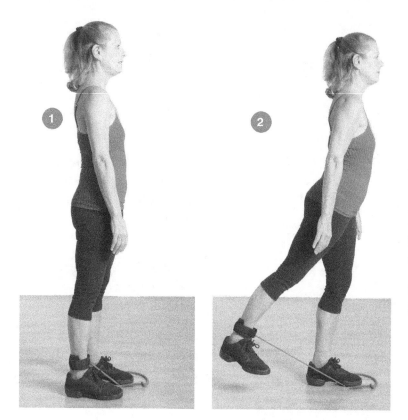

If you have balance issues, hold onto something for stability.

1 Secure the band around each ankle, using either a band with ankle straps or tying an end of the band to each ankle. Adjust the band so that it provides resistance through the full range of motion.

2 Keeping your leg straight, slowly extend your leg backward to engage the butt muscles. Hold for 1–2 seconds.

Slowly return to start position. Repeat, then switch sides.

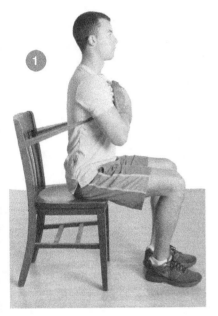

Note that core exercises performed from the floor are superior to this exercise. This exercise is offered for those who cannot perform such core exercises.

1 Sit in a chair with proper posture and place the band behind the upper portion of your chair. Grasp an end of the band in each hand near your shoulders. Adjust your grip on the band until you have your desired resistance.

2 Slowly bend your torso forward. Pause.

Slowly return to start position.

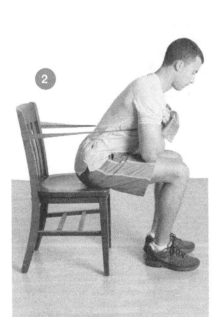

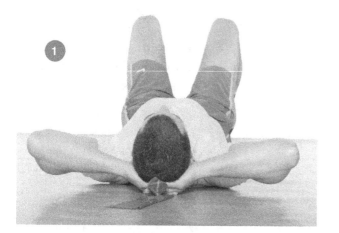

Use a long band for this exercise.

1 Place the band under your tailbone and run it under your spine and head as you lie on your back with your knees bent and feet flat on the floor. Place both hands behind your head and grasp the band.

2 As if doing a traditional half sit-up, tuck your chin to your chest while pressing your lower back into the floor to come up halfway. Hold.

Return to start position.

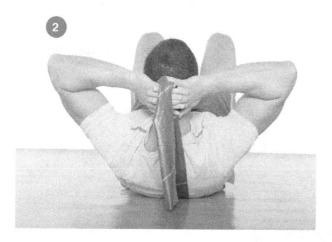

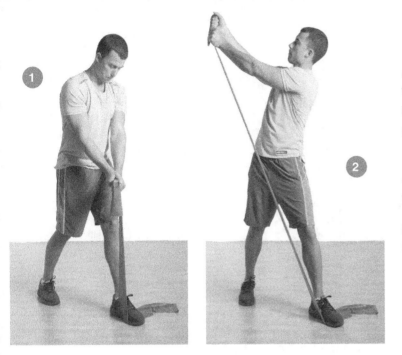

1 Assume a fairly wide staggered stance and step on the band with your left foot. With both hands, grasp the band close to hip height at a point that provides ideal resistance.

2 Rotate your torso diagonally upward to the right, extending your arms upward.

Slowly return to start position. Repeat, then switch sides.

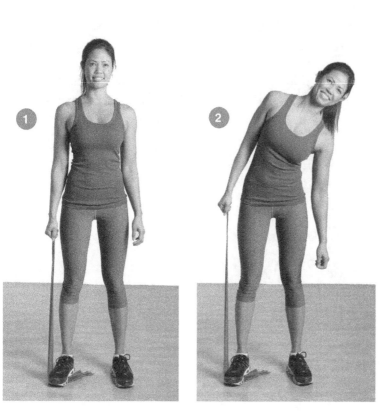

Caution: Be careful if you have arthritis of the spine.

1 Stand with your feet shoulder-width apart and place a band under your right foot. Grasp the band near your right hip with your right hand.

2 Lean your body to the left.

Return to start position. Repeat, then switch sides.

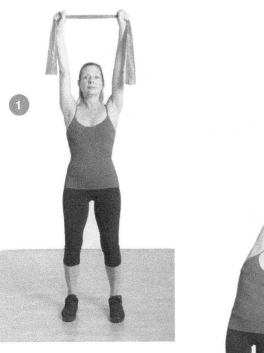

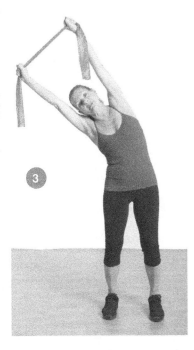

Caution: Be careful if you have arthritis of the spine.

1 Stand with your feet shoulder-width apart and grasp the band in both hands. Raise your arms overhead and pull the band to the sides so that your hands are slightly wider than your shoulders. You should feel some tension in the band.

2 Keeping the tension in the band, lean your body to the left.

3 Return to start position, then lean to the right.

pelvic lift

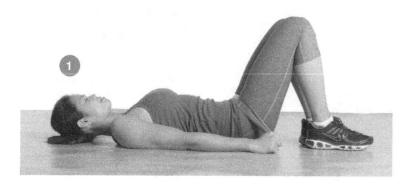

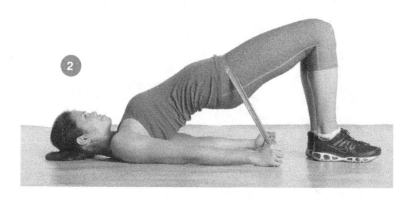

1 Lie on your back. Place the band over your hips and secure it firmly by holding each end of the band with your hands.

2 Slowly lift your hips to a comfortable height. Engage your butt muscles; don't use momentum. Hold for 1–2 seconds.

Return to start position.

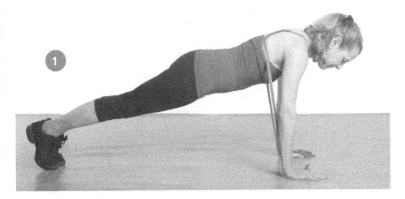

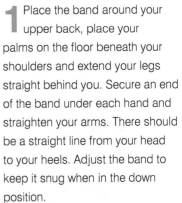

1 Place the band around your upper back, place your palms on the floor beneath your shoulders and extend your legs straight behind you. Secure an end of the band under each hand and straighten your arms. There should be a straight line from your head to your heels. Adjust the band to keep it snug when in the down position.

2 Maintaining a straight spine, slowly lower your chest to the floor.

Extend your arms to return to start position.

MODIFICATION: This can also be done from your knees.

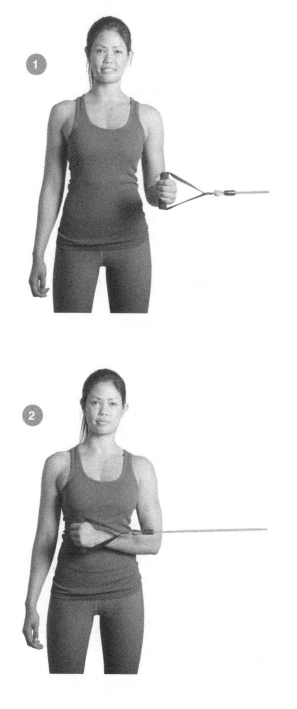

1 Attach the band securely to a stable object (e.g., door knob) at belly button height. With the left side of your body facing the attachment point, grasp the band with your left hand. For a better grip, tie a small knot in the band and then place the band between your ring finger and middle finger with your thumb pointed up. Your left palm should face your body and your left elbow should be bent 90 degrees and next to your ribs. Adjust your distance until you get your desired resistance.

2 Keeping your shoulders back and torso engaged, slowly and mindfully move your left hand to cover your belly button.

Slowly and carefully return to start position. Repeat, then switch sides.

Heavy resistance is not important in this exercise.

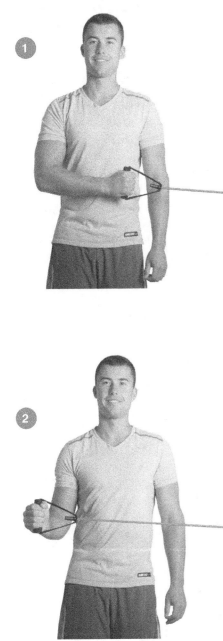

1 Attach the band securely to a stable object (e.g., door knob) at belly button height. With the left side of your body facing the attachment point, grasp the band with your right hand. For a better grip, tie a small knot in the band and then place the band between your ring finger and middle finger with your thumb pointed up. Your right palm should face your body and your right elbow should be bent 90 degrees and next to your ribs. Adjust your distance until you get your desired resistance.

2 Keeping your shoulders back and torso engaged, slowly and mindfully move your right hand out to the side (be careful not to go out too far).

Slowly and carefully return to start position. Repeat, then switch sides.

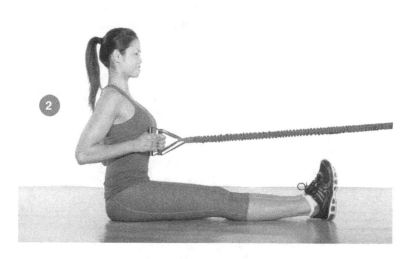

1 Attach the band securely to the bottom of a door or any other stable object. Sit on the floor facing the door then extend your legs straight. Grasp an end of the band in each hand at a location that provides adequate resistance. Keep your torso at roughly 90 degrees.

2 Pull the bands by bending your elbows into your chest.

Slowly allow your arms to return to start position.

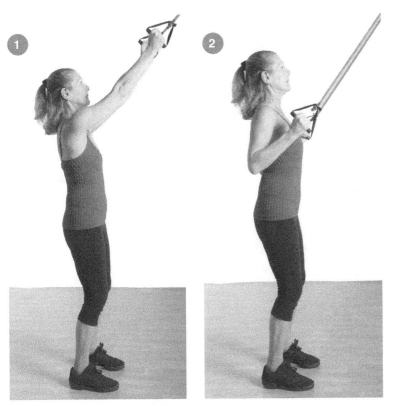

1 Secure the band firmly to the top of a door or something tall and grab an end in each hand. Step backward until the band provides your desired resistance. You may choose to sit on the floor or a chair with your back mostly straight and your arms straight and angled upward.

2 Keeping your elbows close to your ribs, slowly pull the band down toward your chest. Hold for 1–2 seconds.

Slowly release your arms to the start position.

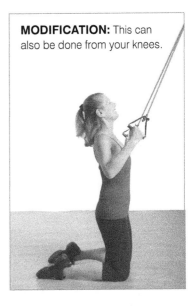

MODIFICATION: This can also be done from your knees.

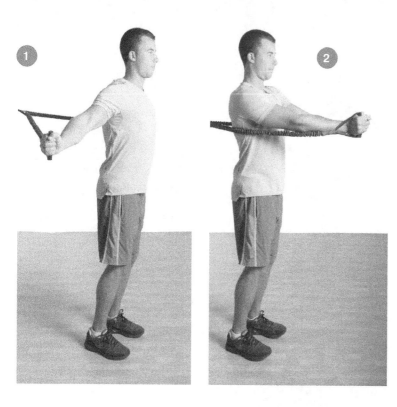

1 Attach the band securely to a door using band straps. With your back to the door, grasp an end of the band in each hand with your arms extended to your sides, palms facing forward.

2 Keeping your arms somewhat straight, bring your arms together in front of your chest, palms facing each other.

Slowly return to start position.

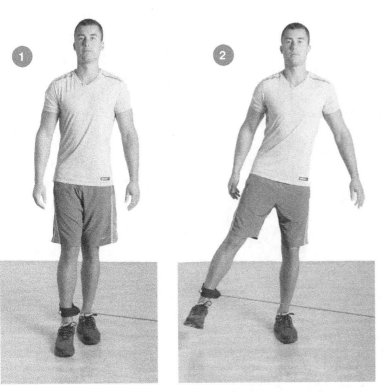

If you have balance issues, hold onto something for stability.

Caution: Avoid this exercise if you have hip problems.

1 Anchor the band firmly at the bottom of a door or similar solid object. Tie the band around your right ankle and then step away from the door with your left side facing it.

2 Slowly move your right leg to the side a comfortable distance.

Repeat, then switch sides.

If you have balance issues, hold onto something for stability.

Caution: Avoid this exercise if you have hip problems.

1 Anchor the band firmly at the bottom of a door or similar solid object. Tie the band around your right ankle and then step away from the door with your right side facing it.

2 Slowly move your right leg in front and across your body to the left.

Repeat, then switch sides.

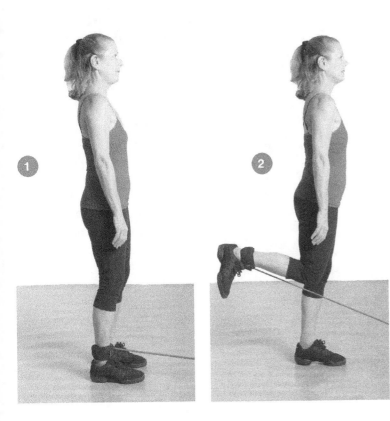

If balance is an issue, you may want to stand near a secure location for assistance.

Caution: Be careful of hamstring cramps.

1 Anchor the band firmly at the bottom of a door or similar solid object. Tie the band around your right ankle and then step away from the door while facing it.

2 Maintaining neutral spine position, slowly curl your right leg. Control the motion in both directions—don't allow the band to determine the speed. Hold for 1–2 seconds.

Slowly lower the leg to start position. Repeat, then switch sides.

94 | **hip extension**   *target: gluteus maximus, hamstrings*

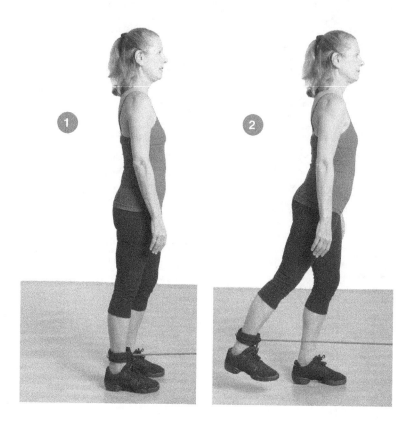

1 Secure the band to a door and then, facing the door, tie one end of the band to your right ankle. Use the door for balance if need be.

2 Keeping your leg straight, slowly extend your leg backward to engage the butt muscles. Hold for 1–2 seconds.

Slowly return to start position. Repeat, then switch sides.

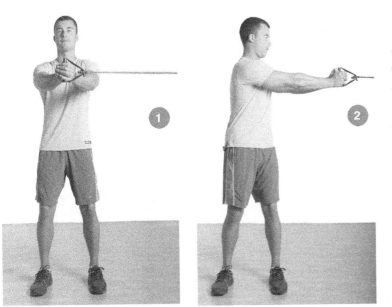

1 Secure the band to a door with the proper strap so that the band is at chest height. While standing with your left side to the door, grab the band with both hands and move away from the door until your arms are fully extended. Stand with your feet shoulder-width apart.

2 Slowly twist to the left and hold for 1–2 seconds.

3 Return to start position.

4 Slowly twist to the right and hold for 1–2 seconds.

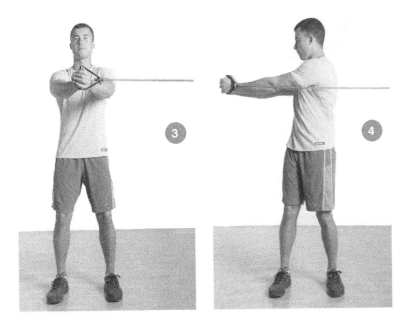

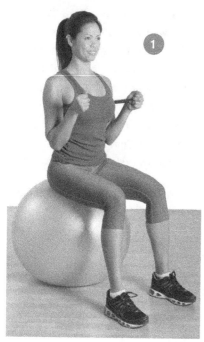

1 Sit properly on the ball and place the band behind your back and under your arms at chest height. Grab the band in each hand at a place that provides ideal resistance.

2 Press the band forward.

Slowly return to start position.

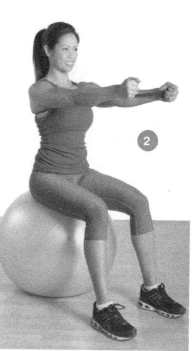

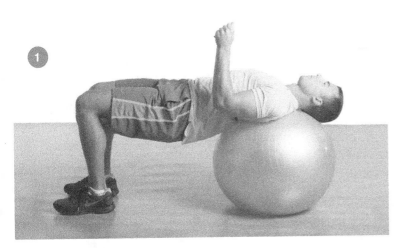

This exercise is extremely tricky and should not be done unless you have experience on a ball.

1 Sit properly on the ball and place the band behind your back and under your arms at chest height. Grab the band in each hand at a place that provides ideal resistance. Now walk your feet forward and slide your butt off the ball until your mid-back is resting on the ball.

2 Press the band to the ceiling until your arms are fully extended.

Slowly control the descent of the band.

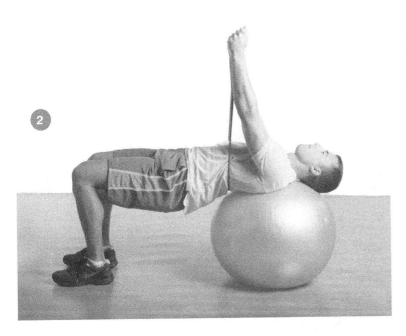

upright flye on ball

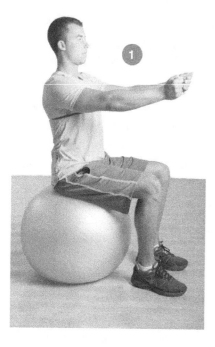

This exercise is extremely tricky and should not be done unless you have experience on a ball.

1 Sit properly on the ball and place the band behind your back and under your arms at chest height. Grab the band in each hand at a place that provides ideal resistance and extend your arms forward.

2 Slowly open your arms to the sides so that they're level with your shoulders.

Bring your arms back to start position.

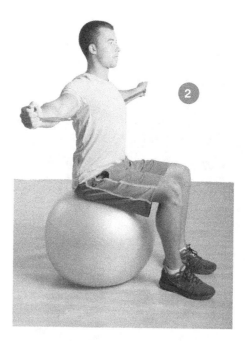

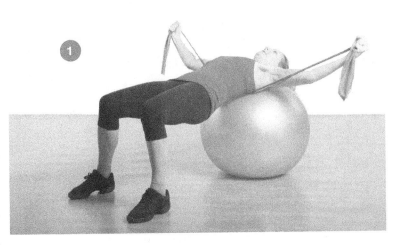

This exercise is extremely tricky and should not be done unless you have experience on a ball.

1 Sit properly on the ball and place the band behind your back and under your arms at chest height. Grab the band in each hand at a place that provides ideal resistance. Now walk your feet forward and slide your butt off the ball until your mid-back is resting on the ball. Slowly lower your arms toward the floor, stopping when they're parallel to the floor.

2 Slowly bring your arms together until your arms are fully extended to the ceiling.

Slowly lower your arms back to start position.

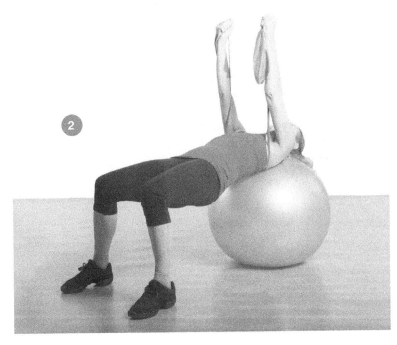

chest press with dumbbells & band

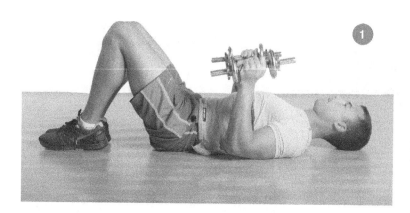

1 Hold a dumbbell in each hand with the ends of the band wrapped around the handles and the band wrapped around your back, under your armpits. Your hands should be at your chest with palms facing each other. Lie on your back with your feet flat on the floor.

2 Press the dumbbells to the ceiling until your arms are fully extended.

Slowly control the descent of the weights back to start position.

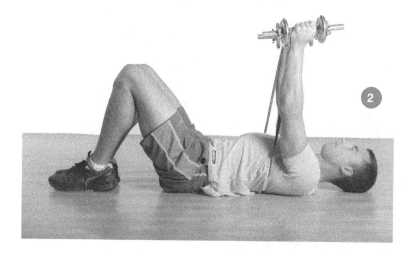

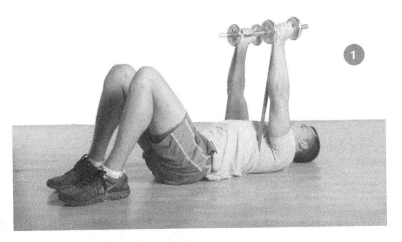

1 Lie on your back with your feet flat on the floor. Hold a dumbbell in each hand with the ends of the band wrapped around the handles and the band wrapped around your back, under your armpits. With your palms facing each other, press the weights to the ceiling. Lie on your back with your feet flat on the floor.

2 Keeping your arms slightly bent, lower your arms to the sides.

Return to start position.

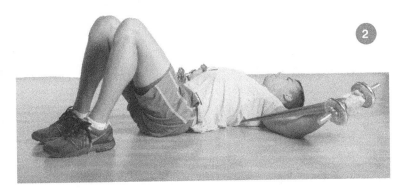

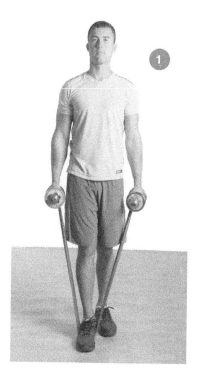

This can be done with one or two hands.

1 Stand on the middle of the band. Hold a dumbbell in each hand with the ends of the band wrapped around the handles. Your arms should be alongside your body, palms facing your body.

2 Keeping your arms straight, slowly raise your arms to the sides no higher than shoulder height.

Slowly return to start position.

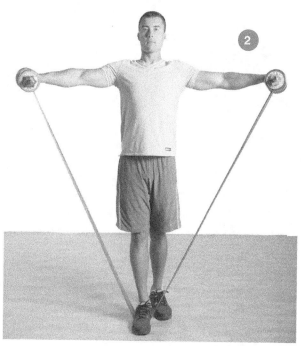

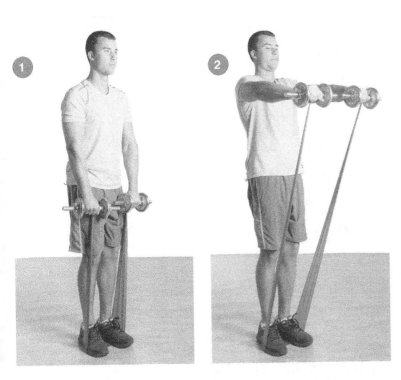

This can be done with one or two hands.

1 Stand on the middle of the band. Hold a dumbbell in each hand with the ends of the band wrapped around the handles. Place your arms in front of your body with your palms facing your thighs.

2 Keeping your arms straight, slowly raise your arms forward no higher than shoulder height.

Slowly return to start position.

biceps curl with dumbbells & band

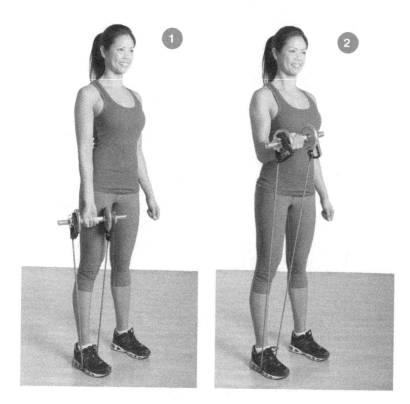

This can be done with one or two hands.

1 Stand with proper posture, feet shoulder-width apart. Hold a dumbbell in your hand with the end of the band wrapped around the handle. Rest your arm along your side.

2 Keeping your elbow next to your torso, slowly curl your hand to your shoulder.

Slowly return to start position. Do not allow the band to determine the speed of descent.

windmill

target: shoulders

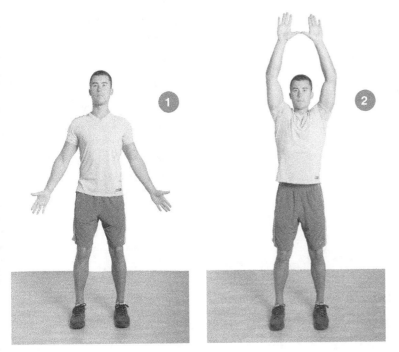

1 Stand with proper posture, your arms at your sides, palms facing forward. Inhale deeply through your nose and slowly raise your arms out to the sides as high as is comfortable. Try to touch your thumbs.

2 Exhale and slowly lower your arms.

Repeat as desired.

SINGLE-ARM VARIATION:
This exercise can also be done one arm at a time.

elbow touch

target: chest, shoulder retractor

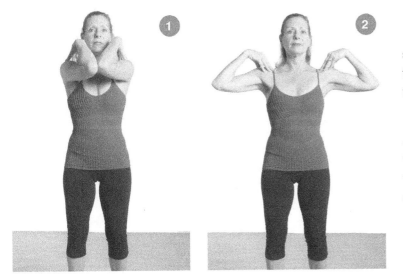

1 Stand with proper posture. Place your hands on your shoulders, elbows pointing forward. Slowly bring your elbows together in front of your body.

2 Bring your elbows back and squeeze your shoulder blades together. Hold for a moment, focusing on opening up your chest.

Bring your elbows back to the starting position and repeat as desired.

1 Stand with proper posture. Inhaling deeply through your nose, slowly lift up your shoulders.

2 Now pull your shoulders back and squeeze the shoulder blades together and down.

3 Exhaling through your lips, drop your shoulders and return to start position.

Repeat as desired.

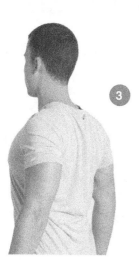

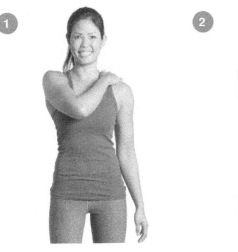
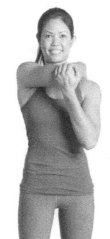

1 Stand with proper posture. Place your right hand on your left shoulder.

2 Place your left hand on your right elbow and gently press your right elbow toward your throat. Hold for a comfortable moment.

Switch sides and repeat.

VARIATION: In Step 2, press your right elbow into your left hand. Hold for a comfortable moment, remembering to breathe. Then release to reach the right hand a little farther back.

lying knee to chest
target: lower back, gluteus maximus

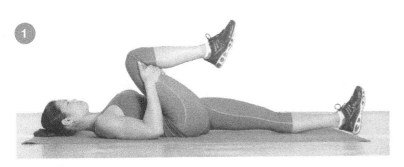

1 Lie on the floor with your legs flat on the floor. Bring your right knee toward your chest and clasp both hands under your right thigh. Hold this position for a comfortable moment, feeling the stretch in the gluteal region.

Release the knee, switch sides and repeat.

sit & reach

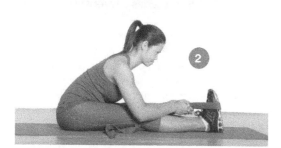

1 Sit on the floor with proper posture and extend both legs out in front of you. Loop a strap around the balls of both feet and hold the ends of the strap in each hand. Inhale deeply through your nose.

2 Now exhale through your lips and gently pull yourself forward by leading with your chest rather than rounding your back. Hold.

Switch sides and repeat.

rear calf stretch

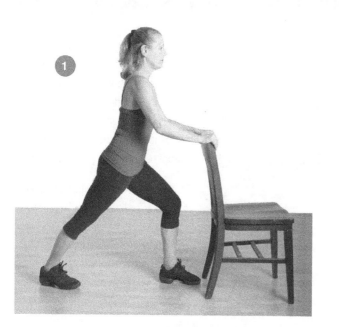

1 Stand behind a chair, placing both hands on the back of the chair. Keeping the heel down, slide your right leg as far back as you can. Bend your left knee until the desired stretch is felt in the calf area. Hold this stretch for a comfortable moment.

Switch sides and repeat.

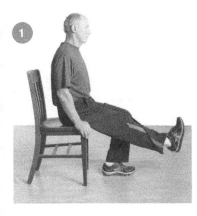

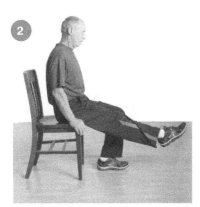

Caution: Do not force your toes in either direction. Be aware that your calf may cramp when extending your toes. Be careful not to tip the chair over.

1 Sit at the edge of a stable chair. Extend your right leg straight out in front of you and lift it off the ground. Point your toes up and hold for several seconds.

2 Point your toes away from you and hold for several seconds.

Repeat a comfortable number of times then switch sides.

twister *target: torso*

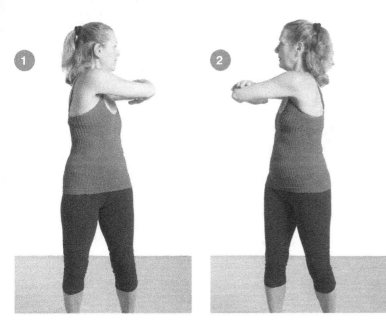

Caution: Be careful if you have lower back problems.

1 Stand with proper posture. Cross your arms in front of your chest and inhale slowly and deeply through your nose. While exhaling through your lips, slowly twist to your left. Hold the position for a comfortable moment and feel the stretch in your torso.

2 Inhale and return to the start position before exhaling and twisting to your right. Hold the position for a comfortable moment and feel the stretch in your torso.

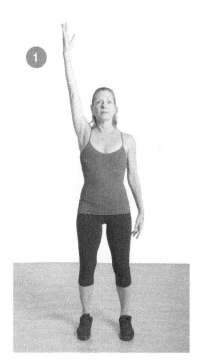

Caution: Be careful if you have lower back pain.

1 Stand with proper posture. Raise your right arm over your head to a comfortable height. Inhale deeply through your nose.

2 Now exhale through your lips and slowly and carefully lean to the left. Once you've leaned over enough to feel a gentle stretch along the right side of your body, hold this position for a comfortable moment.

3 Switch sides and repeat.

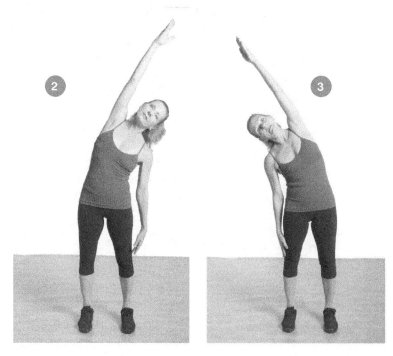

MODIFICATIONS: If your shoulder is stiff, place your hand on top of your head. If raising your arm at all is very painful, just leave your arm alongside your body.

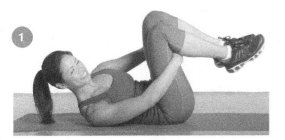

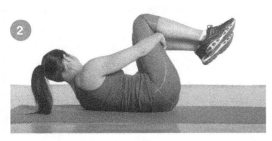

1–2 Lie on a mat and slowly bring both knees toward your chest. Gently reach around both legs and allow your shoulders to lift off the mat. While inhaling deeply through your nose and exhaling through your lips, slowly rock right and left, allowing your side and shoulders to lift off the mat. Enjoy the relaxing feeling.

head tilt — *target: neck*

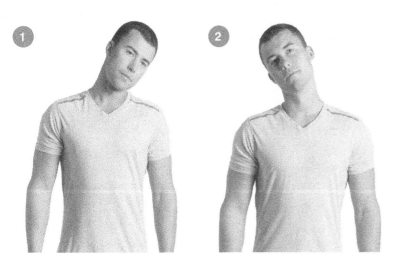

1 Stand with proper posture. While inhaling slowly through your nose, slowly tilt your head toward your left shoulder. Keep your shoulders down and relaxed. Exhale slowly through your lips and hold this position for a moment, feeling the stretch.

2 Now inhale slowly through your nose and slowly tilt your head to your right shoulder. Exhale slowly through your lips and hold this position for a moment, feeling the stretch.

Repeat as desired.

tennis watcher

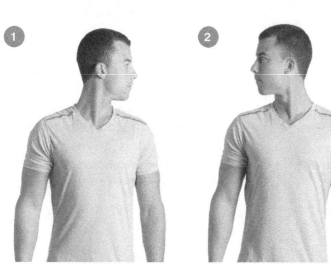

1 Stand with proper posture. While inhaling slowly through your nose, look to your left as far as you can without feeling discomfort. Exhale slowly through your lips and hold this position for a moment, feeling the stretch.

2 Now inhale slowly through your nose and look slowly to the right. Exhale slowly through your lips and hold this position for a moment, feeling the stretch.

Repeat as desired.

index

other karl knopf books

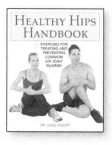

Healthy Hips Handbook
$14.95
Healthy Hips Handbook is designed to help prevent hip problems for some and, for those with existing hip problems, provide post-rehabilitation exercises.

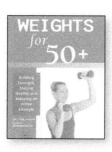

Weights for 50+
$15.95
Weight training is one of the most effective ways to get healthy and fight the physical signs of aging. *Weights for 50+* shows how easy it is for anyone to get started with weights.

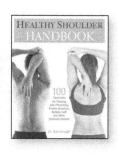

Healthy Shoulder Handbook
$15.95
Includes an overview of shoulder anatomy so anyone can use this friendly manual to strengthen an injured shoulder, identify the onset of a shoulder problem, or better understand injury prevention.

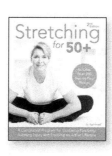

Stretching for 50+
2nd edition
$15.95
Based on the belief that individuals over 50 can do most of the same things as 20- and 30-year-olds, this book shows how to maintain and improve flexibility by stretching.

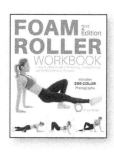

Foam Roller Workbook,
2nd edition
$15.95
Details a comprehensive program for using the foam roller to recover from injury, reverse everyday pain, and stay healthy in the future.

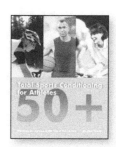

Total Sports Conditioning for Athletes 50+
$14.95
Provides sport-specific workouts that allow aging athletes to maintain the flexibility, strength, and speed needed to win.

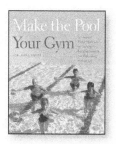

Make the Pool Your Gym
$14.95
Shows how to create an effective and efficient water workout that can build strength, improve cardiovascular fitness, and burn calories.

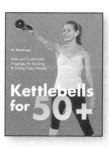

Kettlebells for 50+
$15.95
Offers progressive programs that will improve strength, foster core stability, increase hand-eye coordination, boost mind-body awareness, and enhance sports performance.

To order these books call 800-377-2542 or 510-601-8301, fax 510-601-8307, e-mail ulysses@ulyssespress.com, or write to Ulysses Press, P.O. Box 3440, Berkeley, CA 94703. All retail orders are shipped free of charge. California residents must include sales tax. Allow two to three weeks for delivery.

acknowledgments

Thanks to Peter Pipe for his modification of using a PVC tube as a handle. A special thanks goes to Lily Chou for sharing her insights and knowledge, which significantly improved the outcome of this book. Thanks also go out to the staff at Ulysses Press, whose support made this book possible. Additionally, a giant thank you to the models, Chris Knopf, Mary Gines and Toni Silver. Much appreciation also to the skilled photographic team at Rapt Productions. Lastly, a special thanks goes to my son Chris Knopf for his assistance with this book and to his mother Margaret for allowing me quiet time to work on this project when we could've been doing something fun.

about the author

KARL KNOPF is the author of ten books, including *Core Strength for 50+*, *Kettlebells for 50+*, *Stretching for 50+*, *Foam Roller Workbook*, *Healthy Hips Handbook*, *Healthy Shoulder Handbook* and *Make the Pool Your Gym*. He has been involved with the health and fitness of the disabled and older adults for nearly 40 years. A consultant on numerous National Institutes of Health grants, Knopf has served as advisor to the PBS exercise series *Sit and Be Fit* and to the State of California on disabilities issues. He is a frequent speaker at conferences and has written several textbooks and articles. Knopf coordinates the Fitness Therapist Program at Foothill College in Los Altos Hills, California, and is the director of senior fitness at the International Sports Sciences Association (ISSA).

Printed in the USA
CPSIA information can be obtained
at www.ICGtesting.com
CBHW071811060624
9649CB00005BB/106

9 781612 431710